Research in Clinical Practice

Daron Smith • Dan Wood

Research in Clinical Practice

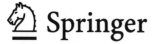 Springer

Daron Smith, MA, BMBch, MD,
FRCS(Urol)
University College Hospital
London
UK

Dan Wood, Phd, FRCS(Urol)
University College Hospital
London
UK

ISBN 978-1-4471-2872-4   ISBN 978-1-4471-2873-1   (eBook)
DOI 10.1007/978-1-4471-2873-1
Springer London Heidelberg New York Dordrecht

Library of Congress Control Number: 2012947023

Printed on acid-free paper

Springer is part of Springer Science+Business Media (www.springer.com)

To our families, who helped and supported us whilst we learned the hard way

Foreword

The ability of society to develop, through the improvement of the health of its members as well as their intellectual and material environment, depends upon the ability of individuals to formulate and test new ideas, based on current knowledge. This notion of research as a developmental tool is therefore open to everyone at all times and applies no less to medicine that any other arena. There is always a tendency to consider research as a preserve of a few individuals who hand down their pearls of wisdom to the majority, who implement them through increasingly narrow, target-orientated processes determined by those in authority. Alternatively, many in professions consider conducting research work as a temporary phase of progression through the apprentice phases to be forgotten when training is completed. However, to sustain and improve the impetus of health-care development requires as wide a participation as possible in the research process – through actual experimentation, education, supervision, or facilitation – whether this is carried out in the workplace or in a more dedicated environment. For those who wish to play an active part in leading the research process, the ability to find a pathway and sustain it is often a daunting and unfamiliar experience. This book by two consultant surgeons who have recently gone down this route is therefore an invaluable tool for the interested participant. It guides the reader to examine what he or she hopes to get from actively participating in research, whom to approach and what questions to ask, the practicalities of actually being able to conduct research in his or her own area of interest, and how to optimize time most effectively. Of equal importance is advice on how to continue this process throughout an entire career, so that once you have joined the research club, there is no escape!

Chris Fry

Foreword

Making Something of Research: "An Introduction?"

Achieving a place at a medical school more or less guarantees you a well-paid and satisfying job for life with a good pension at the end of it. In addition, there are enormous opportunities to become an educationalist, a research scientist, or even a hospital manager (!) either alongside or instead of a clinical career while retaining all of the other benefits. It is, of course, true that any of these career options remain highly competitive, and so each of us must make the most of every opportunity to increase our chances of success in any chosen field. Research is definitely an area where a doctor can enhance their competitiveness with an eye to the future.

In the past, many trainees, particularly on hospital-based career paths, have massaged their CVs by developing a "research profile." The current view suggests that research is best targeted at those who really want to be involved with it and who have a long-term aim to continue to do it or at least be associated with it thereafter. This is not designed to make research an exclusive realm but should rule out any obligation for doctors to go through "a process" if it does not interest them.

There seems little doubt that the best clinical practice is associated with the best teaching in a center in which research is actively being carried out and where excellence is developed by association. Excellence – as Aristotle said – is a habit. It is a way of thinking and a way of acting such that doing the right thing becomes a habit. It is also true that if you are not at the forefront of developing your clinical practice, then you will be left behind by developments in that area. That does not mean that everybody has to be research active but everybody needs to know what research is and how it is done so that they can understand the scientific output in journals and conferences and in casual discussion to be able to discern the truth from the "waffle" (and it is mainly waffle).

Dan Wood and Daron Smith have described here just what one needs to know to be able to start in research and then take a project through it its logical conclusion. It is valuable for those who are about to do research, those who might want to do research, as a refresher for potential clinical supervisors, or those who have no intention of being research active themselves but need to know about "research" as part of their general medical professional development. I have read this book twice and enjoyed it on both occasions. I can certainly recommend it to anybody to read at least once.

Tony Mundy

Preface

This book is designed to be read both by people for whom research is the beginning of an idea and by those who are just embarking on a project. It may also be useful to others, for instance, new supervisors – who are already experienced in their own research but perhaps not in helping others to get started. Even if you have already started in research, there are many useful sections that will also apply to you. The aim is to try to offer help and survival tips as you begin your time in research. Most of the text is based on our own experience, but observations and discussions with many friends and colleagues suggest that the difficulties people have are similar and probably avoidable.

We have no stronger claim to be experts on the process of research than anyone else. While our individual experiences were quite different, we had the benefit of working alongside some very bright, committed, and extremely supportive people during our time as research fellows. Largely through the support of clinical trainers, supervisors, and the understanding of families, we have been fortunate to continue with some aspects of research.

The original idea for this book was borne out of the day to day frustrations and near misses that were a normal pattern – certainly in the early days of our research. Many of those people with whom we have worked will recognize parts of this book as it includes many ideas that we have freely discussed over the years – in many ways, the only way this book could be written is by having listened to and combining the experience of those people we have been lucky enough to work with. As time passes, it appears that many fellows are allowed to repeat the same mistakes – this has become clearer with time as we see more people go through the same process. Time in research is a huge chunk of an individual's life. It requires significant energy – both professional and emotional, financial commitments from grant giving bodies, financial sacrifice (compared with the salary of a clinician), and a huge commitment from a department and supervisor. In the past, we have all undertaken this without a guide or framework – it is no wonder that we all encountered such difficulties. We hope that this book will offer some useful suggestions of ways around these pitfalls.

It was put to us before starting research that it is far worse to have done research and have little or nothing to show for it than not to do it at all. This remains largely true. There continue to be many problems with research that will not change imminently. There will never be "enough" money, and as long as there is no official regulation from the grant bodies or colleges for clinicians, anyone can take on a research fellow and offer supervision. The outcome of research is rarely checked (apart from indirectly – by training committees, etc.) and it is still true that huge numbers of projects undertaken are not written up. Research has frequently been a means to an end for trainees to achieve points and make themselves more competitive in the application process for clinical jobs. It remains true that points can often be gained by having registered for and completed a higher degree. If this is your only motivation, you can expect increasing frustration as you encounter the inevitable trials and tribulations of research – if you lack a genuine interest or enthusiasm for your work, it will drive down the quality of what you achieve.

In competitive specialties, getting an edge over your peers can be difficult, and research may be one way of demonstrating commitment and an ability to work independently. However, in specialties where research has become so common as to be a virtual necessity, there will be examples of people who undertake a project purely to fill a gap in their CV. This is not a failing on their part as they often have little option – although the system is changing to avoid this. Research postings should be regarded as precious commodities, not something given away as an interim post. If you are taking on a project or looking at doing research, then consider why you are doing it. If you are doing it because you have to – think again. Can you achieve your objective in other ways? If you find a desire to do research later because you want to, then it will be better for all concerned.

Once you have committed to the idea of research, careful planning is vital for success. The aim of this book is to help you through some aspects of that planning: rather than being a comprehensive guide to your project, it aims to help you anticipate problems and find solutions before they become a major disruption to your work.

At the end of each chapter, you will find a short, summary table giving the key points, giving you an outline of the chapter and, in some instances, acting as a checklist.

Whatever research you are undertaking, we hope that it is an exciting and enjoyable time for you. If you achieve this, then you and your supervisor have done a good job and you will have made a contribution to the knowledge base of your subject.

Consider the Context

At the time of writing, countless individuals have undertaken research in order to fill a box on their CV and make themselves more competitive in the job market. This outmoded approach is expensive and, when research is not completed, frankly wasteful. The authors hope to see this will continue to be regarded as an old-fashioned view of research – and with the increasing development of Academic Clinical Fellow and Clinical Lectureships, fully expect that it will.

Until then, the aim of this book is to help introduce an individual to research and guide them to overcome the early pitfalls. It should be recognized by every reader that we do not see research as an isolated event in a doctor's life but rather that it becomes something to build on as a part of career progression. Ideally, you will go on to apply for further grants, take on research fellows, and encourage good research projects of your own as a supervisor. This can only come if you maximize your own opportunities. We hope that this book will go some way to encouraging you to do this, and perhaps, as you read on, you should consider the book in this context too.

London   DW & DS
April 2013

Contents

Contributors

Hashim Ahmed, MRCS, BM, BCh, BA(Hons)
Division of Surgery and Interventional Science,
University College London, London, UK

**Jo Cresswell, MBBS, BMedSCi,
PhD, FRCS(Urol)**
Department of Urology, James Cook Hospital,
Middlesbrough, UK

**Niki Thiruchelvam, MBBS, BSc, MRCS MD,
FRCS (Urol) FEBU**
Department of Urology,
Addenbrookes Hospital, Cambridge, UK

Chapter 1
Setting Up a Project

Research n. systematic investigation into and study of materials and sources etc. in order to establish facts and reach new conclusions.
Oxford English Dictionary.

See Table 1.1 for key points of the chapter.

As a clinician undertaking research, your future career will depend on the outcome. This is a positive statement and should serve as a motivation. If you are able to find a good supervisor and a project that interests and excites you, you will work hard at it. This will stimulate a genuine interest, if it did not already exist. A combination of all these factors will lead to you to perform a thorough investigation – establishing facts for yourself and developing the ability to reach your own, new conclusions (see the definition above).

Under these circumstances, it will be easier to achieve your career goals. You will have publications to your name, possibly a thesis and your supervisor will be happy to reinforce your reputation as a hard worker that people should listen to. This does not mean that you will be pigeon-holed into an academic career, but it may remain an option if you choose it.

D. Smith, D. Wood, *Research in Clinical Practice*,
DOI 10.1007/978-1-4471-2873-1_1,
© Springer-Verlag London 2013

Taking on a research project will offer a whole range of opportunities including the development of technical and personal skills, publication of work and national and international travel to present your work. You may undertake it with a view to establishing an academic career for some your time in research will exceed all expectations, your interest and focus may begin to develop during this time.

Overall failure in research comes in various forms and is probably accompanied by a number of factors but generally has one aspect at the core: the individual. You will already have realized the importance of self-motivation – you may survive your time in research without this, but you will struggle to make a success of it. You will encounter many problems as part of your research – even in the best lab with a well-planned project. It is the very nature of what you are doing – to solve problems. Somebody with a lack of drive may not be able to see those problems through – or they will eventually be worn down by them and their project will flounder.

In order to perform good research, three factors are important – the project, the individual, and the supervisor – in no particular order! This chapter gives a brief introduction to these areas allowing for expansion later in the book.

Choosing a Project

Your reasons for doing research start here. If you have reached a senior level and wish to perform research, you may well have a specific interest or area that you wish to develop. There is no doubt that this is an advantage. You will probably have a significant knowledge base in the area, may have had a long-term association with your proposed supervisor, and will, perhaps, have begun provisional planning sometime beforehand. In this situation, your established enthusiasm and knowledge will be a great asset.

In recent years, those undertaking research have tended to be more junior and are, therefore, less likely to have had such a clear idea about what they want to do. This was certainly true before the advent of Modernising Medical Careers when research was often done as a stepping-stone between SHO and SpR posts. Prior to this most research was undertaken by senior registrars – usually with a clear interest.

More recently still, there has been a far greater development of systematic opportunities for research – such as the creation of Academic Clinical Fellowships (ACFs). This shows a clearer investment in academic pathways for some. Some of these fellowships will result in out of program research blocks for a higher degree, offering trainees a post with 25 % of their time dedicated to formulating a research project. Following this, individuals wishing to continue in research would be expected to have gained a research grant to fund a higher degree and subsequently competitive entry to a clinical lectureship post.

For any junior doctor entering research, either during an out of program experience or as an ACF, the selection of the right project is a difficult, but crucial decision. It is therefore vital to take expert advice on how to approach a research project. First of all, is it what you want to do? Would you rather apply for a "standard" National Training Number – could you learn and achieve by publishing on the job? It is a mistake to think that dedicated time in research is an easy option – your day-to-day timetable may be less arduous, or at least be more flexible, but you will find pressures of a different sort. If you think you have to do some form of research but are not sure that a dedicated project is for you – consider one of the taught MSc courses. As an ACF you will fast discover that 1 day/week is hardly any time at all if meaningful achievements are to be made – you will have to focus this time and formulate a good project, get a grant and plan to move to a period of full-time research.

Many people would get all they need out of research by learning about methodology, understanding data analysis, and an in-depth look at the basic science around their own area. This summarizes the outline of a generic MSc course – there is a wide choice of content, and these courses are usually well structured. For example, many such courses require the writing of a thesis based on a smaller-scale research project. They are a very good way of getting a lot out of the research environment without having to stop clinical work – although there are some full-time courses. They are also hard work and require a lot of input, so should not be undertaken lightly. For those prepared to put in an appropriate effort, the outcome will be a feeling of success and a very solid grounding in their subject.

The Individual

One should not overanalyze a situation, but it is important to be honest with yourself about why you are considering research. Have you envisaged a glittering academic career, are you looking to gain CV points, or have you run out of other options? Those clinicians who do well at research are a self-selected, highly motivated group. They enter the frame aware of pressure to complete a project within a set period, and their drive is to achieve exactly that. If you are not in this category, you need to look far deeper than whether research is right for you but examine if you have chosen the correct career path altogether.

There is a discussion regarding the value of research to a clinician in his or her career. Some would seek to remove it as a differentiator in the appointment process and that may end up as the case. However, this would go against successful examples of appointment processes in other places, such as the USA and Australasia, where academic success continues to give weight to candidates' scoring. It is possible that a continued resistance to recognize research will lead to a reduction in the number of people undertaking it in a formal setting – at least, temporarily. It raises the concern that in many cases research is undertaken solely to fill a box on an application form and hence the overall motivation along with the outcome is often poor. For those people who do good research, it is more common that they have a particular interest in looking deeply into their subject. When good research is completed, it demonstrates a committed individual who is able to show initiative and independence. Therefore, even if those charged with appointing doctors remove research as a criterion for short-listing, it is likely that those individuals who are interested will still pursue it. Therefore, those people who enter research will continue to show a level of commitment and independence that will stand them in good stead for appointment to a job at any level. In essence undertaking research will not do you any harm – provided you are keen and motivated to complete it.

Your Supervisor

Your supervisor will play a crucial role in your research and its success (or not) and will act as your lifeline. In the best organized departments, you are likely to form only a small part of your supervisor's overall research strategy. It is important to remember this – while your research project will become central to your world, your supervisor may have many other projects running at the same time. Yours can only ever be equal in importance to those others – try to remember that in your dealings with your supervisor and the rest of the lab team.

When you are deciding on a project, you may meet a number of potential supervisors; try to keep a list of things that interest you in mind so that you are able to give them some information about projects that might suit you. It would be unusual to expect your early thoughts to be so defined that you arrive with an unwavering desire to measure transmembrane sodium flux in cells from the frog retina or equally subspecialized topic. However, you may have encountered a clinical problem that you would like to investigate from either a clinical or a basic science perspective. This may not be where you finally decide your project lies, but it is a useful starting point for a conversation.

When making these decisions, it is important to try to maintain a broad-minded approach. Try to consider your options from a number of angles, such as, what projects are available, what projects would interest you, and what projects are likely to fit with your future career plan?

It is often helpful to have an idea about a 5-year plan, i.e. what you plan to do next and how you plan to get there. This should not be something that you feel you have to stick to rigidly, but it does give you some objectives and a sense of purpose. If you change, or adapt, it is not a problem. It is often much easier to cope with threats and problems with a change in objectives – than having to start from scratch.

When reading through subsequent sections of this book, try to remember that your research commitment is about developing an understanding and furthering knowledge in a new area. Overall, this is exciting but do not expect the day-to-day dealings of that to always to be rewarding, but by putting yourself in the right place with the right people and working toward a defined end point, you stand a chance of having both an enjoyable and successful time in research.

You must look to leave research with additional maturity, research acumen, some technical research skills, publication(s), and a thesis. This is a tall order, and your focus must be tailored toward achieving these objectives (Table 1.1).

Table 1.1 Introductory points

The choice of project is a crucial decision – seek and act on expert advice early
Decide between a whole time out of program project versus "on the job" research, perhaps with an Academic Clinical Fellowship, or consider a structured MSc
Recognize that your supervisor is the likely key to success (read on!)

Chapter 2
Choosing a Project, Location, and Supervisor

See Table 2.1 for chapter summary.

The location of your research will be fundamental in determining its success. There are several aspects to selecting a location, and these will be considered in the next few pages.

In choosing where you decide to work, there are three main issues that you need to consider.

1. Subject – what area do you wish to research – you may not know precisely, but you should have a broad idea as to what your interest could be, or might develop into.
2. Supervisor – having thought about a sensible subject area, you will need to think about who you want to work for. Different labs will have different setups – and these vary over time. Some may be happy for you to join the lab and work on a project providing you have or can bring some funding. Others may have already allocated funding and be seeking applicants to fill a post.
3. Money – nobody likes to discuss money but you will need to. If you are just about to look into a project, you will need to know on what basis you and the project are going to be funded and can be sure that this will be sustained until your project can be completed.

D. Smith, D. Wood, *Research in Clinical Practice,*
DOI 10.1007/978-1-4471-2873-1_2,
© Springer-Verlag London 2013

Choosing Your Subject

The definition of an expert is someone who knows more and
more about less and less! Anon.

The trend for taking up research has changed completely
over the last decade or so, and with the development of MMC
and other changes it may alter further – or revert to previous!
Research used to be the realm of senior registrars who had
already established an area of clinical practice that they were
aspiring toward, and therefore the subject of their research
would be more obvious. In an ever developing world of
research, there may be a return to this.

In recent times, attempts to change the registrar's appointment process and selection criteria have often questioned the
role of research as a means of differentiating applicants. Yet
there is no question about the need for continued development of medical and scientific knowledge, and therefore good
research will always be required and valued. It is also true
that achievement in research is an excellent and well-estab-
lished way to demonstrate both excellence and commitment
to a specialty. The 2008 debacle that was [1]MTAS (Medical
Training Application Service) was symptomatic of constant
change – while many changes are for the better, some may
cause massive distress and disruption. Despite change it is
important to maintain a positive focus for success – the same
rules will be applied to all, and if you are good, your chances
of success remain high. It seems vital that anyone planning a
long-term career in a specialty will need to be committed and
a successful appointment process will have to take account of
this. Similarly, entry to such programs should remain a privi-
lege that can be attained on merit alone; hence, excellence
must also be demonstrable. Why mention this? While changes

---

[1] MTAS – Medical Trainees Appointment System – was a centralized,
electronic appointment process for junior doctors that was used in 2008.
It was universally acknowledged as having a number of failures that lead
to difficulties for junior doctors looking for appointments at the time. It
was part of a process examined in the Tooke Report.

in the system have shown many weaknesses, they demonstrated the importance of essential and desirable criteria in an application process. Anybody applying for a job must, by definition, have all the essential criteria – therefore candidates can only be separated by additions to these – that is, including the desirable criteria. It is certainly true that making it desirable for candidates to have collected 50 coins from the Roman Empire in order to get a job will mean that the truly committed individual will turn up with 100 fine examples. This somewhat ridiculous example illustrates that in a competitive environment, people will always seek to separate themselves from the pack, and achieving more than your peers – for example, through better research – is one way of doing this.

Undertaking research earlier in a career may make it more difficult for an individual to know what to investigate. Many worry about pigeon-holing themselves too early – but if you are interested in committing to academia, you will have to take the plunge at some point. Research does not necessarily confine you to an area for life, but if you have relevant research behind you, it can only be an advantage. In some ways, the exact subject of your project is less important than your developing an understanding of the scientific method and research process. The grounding you will have obtained from your research will allow your future career to follow a different scientific direction if you do adjust your particular area of practice later in your training. Of course, it helps if you are already genuinely interested in the subject as this will maintain your motivation throughout the project. The caveat of changing direction such that your research does not relate to the rest of your career leaves the onus on you to demonstrate that your research training has allowed you to achieve the skills to maintain a research interest in your final area of practice. It is therefore much the better to select a subject area that you expect to maintain and develop an interest in throughout your career.

In order to approach this important decision, start by trying to break things up into major categories. For instance, do you want to do clinical or nonclinical research; do you want to look at areas involving oncology or not? The more categories that you consider, the more this process will begin to narrow down your choices and help you to make up your mind. Nothing is irreversible at this stage – so if a deeper look leads you to change your plans, this will not matter – better now than later on… If you are completely stuck for direction, write down everything that interests you from stamp collecting to glacier abseiling – looking at your life in the broadest sense may help you to see which way to turn for this decision or it may put you off altogether!

The next step is to try to think about the advantages and disadvantages of everything you have on your list – for instance, with clinical research you may be just part of a huge project that is running for years – you have to ask what will you gain; will there be any papers for you to write and will you complete a credible thesis? However, you are likely to be able to maintain some of your clinical skills and may even learn new ones that will stand you in good stead for the future, and there may be additional papers for a number of years that will continue to have your name on them. If you sign up to work in a laboratory, you are more likely to benefit from an education in scientific method and the time to develop your research in new directions. These are aspects to your career that might be extremely difficult to acquire at any other time. However, you need to understand that this will be a period of sometimes frustrating work, learning new techniques, working among new colleagues (many of them non-medical), and sometimes isolated from the clinical world. Essentially, this remains a very individual decision. You are not usually bound by the same constraints of application for a clinical job. The majority of supervisors will understand and indeed encourage the need to look at other possibilities in order that you take on exactly the right research project for you. In selecting the subject, you should be prepared to do some leg work. This means visiting laboratories or departments, chatting to supervisors and, ideally, their current and even previous research fellows, and discovering what a project might involve. It is worth doing your own literature search and finding out which names appear to be important. This will also help with familiarizing yourself with current important topics in your prospective subject area.

When you are close to making a decision, talk to friends and possibly your current clinical or educational supervisor (or another who you feel will give you honest advice). It is easy to get carried away with an idea and not see the pitfalls. In the end, nobody can make the decision for you, but you may hear things that you had not thought of before which will help to clarify your decision making.

Supervision

There are many stories of people who started research and were buried in a basement on a back street with no money, no teaching, and no support. There are also stories of those who have been well supported throughout their research. In both groups, there are successes and failures. In the first, success comes down to a degree of luck and a lot of hard work on the part of the individual. In the second group, your hard work is still essential, but your need for luck is greatly reduced. For a project to be a success, you need a combination of support, hard work, and luck. It is obviously better to build your foundations on the basis of good support and hard work, rather than hoping for good luck, although a bit of this definitely helps! Clearly, the key element to your success is your supervisor. With his or her leadership, the rest of the essential elements will fall into place.

In the University of London, approximately 50 % of theses (from clinicians) enrolled for are never submitted. This is close to theft: in effect, you have signed up to produce a piece of work – you may even have been paid to do so – and if you fail to show any meaningful output, you will have defaulted on your side of the bargain. In other walks of life, this would be termed "a breach of contract." This has a huge impact on research in general – grant-giving bodies will look less favorably on you and your supervisor in the future. There is a lot of time, effort, and money that is wasted, and it may well have a detrimental effect on your career progression.

Universities also view different types of research degree differently. PhD students will find a strong tendency for universities to adhere closely to a fairly rigid set of rules. This can be a major advantage as it offers a structure to your time and will usually require you to complete a logbook and to achieve various milestones. The approach to an MD can be less rigid and will depend on both the university and your supervisor. In either case universities will often have courses available to graduate students such as statistics, presentation, management, teaching, etc.; these may be very useful in both content and adding weight to your CV. Discuss these aspects with your supervisor and any fellows; it may help you to gauge the environment within a prospective institution.

Choosing the Right Supervisor

The following sections cover five areas in making this choice. You can find out many of these by asking around, especially current and previous research fellows. Ask them how they got on, what happened when they hit a problem, and how were they taught about the department and relevant techniques during their project. Also ask about the support available while writing up – how long did it take for the supervisor to return their thesis and how quickly did they correct drafts of papers or theses?

Presence

It is fantastic and exciting to work for internationally renowned figures. However, you need to be realistic if you get such an opportunity, and close questioning in the unit is vital. Often units like this run on two levels; the great woman (or man!) contributes with energy, ideas, some funding, and an overall vision for the unit and will provide detailed input when possible. Often the day-to-day running of such a unit is provided by a right-hand man (or woman!). If you are lucky enough to have an opportunity to work in such an environment, you need to understand how it operates. It would be pointless to work in circumstances where everything you do day to day is according to the right-hand man, but when the boss arrives, they change everything to their own way – you will simply end up caught between the two and achieve nothing. The same is true if you have both a scientific and clinical supervisor who do not agree on the overall direction of the project. You can only find out these details by asking current fellows – so do ask as many as you can.

If you look likely to spend large periods of time without any supervision, then consider looking elsewhere. Research is hard work – you will definitely encounter problems, and if your supervisor is constantly away presenting or teaching you risk suffering constant delays to your progress.

In summary, it does not matter how good or famous your supervisor is (or was); if they are not there, they cannot supervise you. In some units, you have to have two supervisors, and this may help to solve this problem, but you must check with others how this works, in practice, before you take it on.

Approachable

This is too fundamental to dwell on. As clinicians, we have all worked for consultants who were utterly unapproachable – for various reasons. This is tolerable for 6 months when doing a clinical job, and direct exposure can be fairly dilute.

In a research setting, you need to be able to approach your supervisor and ask them the most simple (and sometimes even stupid!) questions. You will have times when you simply do not understand very basic things, especially at the beginning of your project, when making a positive start is extremely important to get you heading in the right direction. This is a vital element as it will help you to build momentum and motivation for the rest of your time in research. If you cannot clarify a fundamental issue, the rest will remain much more difficult. When you are sizing up a position, you need consider your potential personal relationship with your supervisor as one of the most important factors in your decision making.

Grant Applications

In our view there are four types of supervisor when it comes to grant applications, and it is, arguably, one factor that distinguishes the wheat from the chaff.

Type 1 – "Most members of the team do some casualty locums, or RMO work on the side, which seems to cover costs. Just let me know your details so we know who to invoice for the bench fees"

Type 2 – "As the clinical fellow we expect you to provide cover for clinics on Wednesday, Thursday and Friday. Monday and Tuesday are you own, unless you are on call or one of the others is on leave."

Type 3 – "Well done very pleased to have you on board. Here are the details of some groups who sometimes give grants. Let me see your applications when you've done them so I can check the grammar and put my name on it."

Type 4 – "Thank you for showing an interest. We need between 6 months and one year to help you get some money together. Let me have the details of your current salary and together we can set about finalizing the details of the project and applying for grant money."

Clearly these are exaggerated examples, once again, to make a point. In the case of type 1, you will spend your time doing night shifts and weekend work which, even with your best efforts, will detract from your time in research and make it harder to focus on your project. It may be acceptable to start your project in this situation when you know that there is a grant that is due to start funding in a short time. There are no guarantees that you will get a grant (the hit rate is about 1 in 5), so if you do not have anything definite, you may end up doing this for some time.

Type 2 is perhaps the most dangerous situation. You will be pulled in both directions and feel guilty when you do not fulfill your obligations. These may become increasingly clinical and when you come to discuss how your research is going – who do you think will take the blame for not getting the project further off the ground?

Type 3 is enthusiastic, but probably with unrealistic expectations, either for the project itself or the chance of getting it funded. Gaining a grant is very difficult: you will need help, support, and a huge amount of guidance to get your first grant. If you do not have this, you will struggle (of course there are stories of success, and while huge personal endeavor will have been important, luck will have played a big part too). You may wish to have a go at drafting the grant yourself, but be prepared to use all the help you can get to refine it. This means that you will need to plan long in advance of the submission date.

Type 4 is ideal. Your prospective supervisor should be advising you with realistic time frames so that you can compete for and set up a grant prior to your arrival. If you are very fortunate, all this will have been done before you get there (but regrettably this is very rare). You need about a year to set things up this way, but there is a great deal of satisfaction in having been involved right from the start.

Knowledge

Getting grants and writing publications require a tremendous insight into an area if they are to be successful. Your supervisor may well have a number of Medline publications to their name to attest to their knowledge. It is reasonable and indeed sensible to look these up. This will help you on two levels:

- You will prove to yourself that your prospective supervisor does have relevant expertise in your field of inquiry field.
- You will have discovered a ready-made source of background reading.

It is very useful to know what the current fellows say – are they helped with answering questions and given guidance, or are they left to their own devices?

Track Record

This is implicit in the previous point. In addition to checking your supervisor's own publication record, what is their record on getting fellows to complete a thesis and how many of the fellows got a grant while working in their department?

There is probably not a dream supervisor who scores perfectly by this guide (although there are some who come close!). Analyzing each facet separately will allow you to identify the strengths and weaknesses of a situation. It may be that you are confident in some of your personal strengths that might allow you to accept and cover certain other deficits by yourself.

Money

There are very few grant-maintained posts that are ready-made for you to step into. This means you need to allow time before you start to apply for and get a grant. You will have done very well if you are successful with your first application – do not be disheartened by initial failures – as we have said above the success rate is about one in five.

You will maximize your chances of success by involving yourself early on with a good supervisor. A good unit has probably become so by attracting lots of grant money so they may have slightly better hit rate on the basis of previous experience.

Before you apply for a research post, you should have details of your current salary available and ensure that you can continue your pension scheme contributions if you wish to.

In reality, many people are already coming to the end of a job when they start to think of research. The ideal situation is to give yourself another 6–9 months grace by getting an interim clinical post (which will provide useful added experience to your CV and may even adjust the focus of your research ideas) rather than rush to start a project with no money. This is better because you will not have to scratch around for locum work and can get straight into your project when the time comes. It also means that you have time to formulate a plan before you start which is a much more sensible basis on which to begin than arriving on day one with a blank sheet of paper. It is not always possible to do this; hence, some people do start with grant applications in progress, relying on interim funding on a more ad hoc basis, either by arranging thier own locums or by providing clinical support for the unit attached to the research institute. The obvious drawback to this is that if your grant application fails, you are committed to funding yourself until the next round of grant applications – or facing a delay until the money eventually comes through. During that period you are losing valuable time that you could be using to concentrate on your project. In addition, you will be astonished by the cost of consumables. Even if you can find your own salary with locums, you will need the support of your supervisor and research unit to cover the cost of consumables until you have your own funding to pay for these. This must be discussed and agreed before you arrive.

Finally, even though a 2- or 3-year period spent on a project sounds like a long time, you want to leave your time in research with your data complete and your thesis written up; otherwise, you will struggle to finish it from a clinical job. If you have to spend days away doing locum work, you are less likely to achieve this.

In summary (see Table 2.1), set everything up to be as favorable as it can be, choosing the location that offers you the subject you prefer. Do the leg work first and spend time

Table 2.1 Supervisors key attributes

Presence – they must be there and available
Approachable – you must be able to ask them stupid questions – you will need to
Grant applications – you need help with writing grants
Knowledge – they must know the subject area you are involved in
Track record – setting out with a complete newcomer is a risky strategy

talking to prospective supervisors. The responsibility to check and choose the correct post is yours. Aim to set up finances before you start – time is precious and you cannot afford to waste it. Investing this amount of effort before you actually start your project gives you the best chance of success.

Chapter 3
Choosing a Degree

See Table 3.1 for chapter summary.

If you are undertaking a research project, you should be clear with yourself, your supervisors, and your prospective employers as to your aims. Those aims may change for good reason, but you must begin with a specific objective in mind. It is sensible that within these considerations you will come to a decision about which research degree you wish to register for.

Undertaking a short project to write a paper is a perfectly reasonable objective, but do ensure that everyone is clear about your goal – do not, for instance, claim that you are off to work for a doctorate when you have no intention of doing so. If you are aiming to complete a higher degree, look carefully at your options. It is important to check the regulations of your local university or the one to which you will be registered. Most commonly your choices will be between the Master of Science (MSc), Doctorate of Medicine (MD or DM, which can only be undertaken if you have a previous medical degree), and Doctorate of Philosophy (PhD – which can be undertaken by anybody subject to acceptance by a university).

D. Smith, D. Wood, *Research in Clinical Practice,*
DOI 10.1007/978-1-4471-2873-1_3,
© Springer-Verlag London 2013

Master of Science (MSc)

In many ways this will present you with the most choices. The principle of an MSc is a taught course with a research element. This means that you will receive a dedicated lecture course covering the area of interest for your degree – examples include surgical science, education, clinical pharmacology, and many, many others. This may be delivered on a full-time or part-time (day-release) basis. You need to check the flexibility of the course and the availability of places – in some courses, limited places may mean that there is a waiting list, although universities will have a motivation to take you on as you will attract (i.e., pay) fees and if you are successful then you will have been a positive asset for them. It is crucial that you establish whether, for instance, a part-time course is likely to fit in with your current employment. You will really cause trouble for yourself if you sign up for a course that you have not previously agreed with your employer and for which you will not then be released. This will result in you wasting your time, losing your fee, as well as irritating your boss and your referee.

Once again start by doing your homework – look at courses, their cost, their location, and the time commitment required. This information is now readily available over the Internet and is probably not much more than a couple of evenings work. Talk to your current consultant at the planning stage – what do they think? Will they support you and your plans? They have a responsibility to ensure that the departmental service commitment is maintained – how will your work be covered? You may need to talk to the clinical managers (ideally with your consultant present – hence, the importance of having their support from the outset). Also talk to your educational tutor and try to assess what they think it will offer for you in terms of your future career. If they think it will be of no advantage, that does not, necessarily, mean you should not proceed. If you are keen to undertake this for your own reasons, you should do so. Research is a personal goal; those motivated by CV filling intent as a sole objective will struggle much more than those with a wider view.

Doctorate of Medicine (MD or DM)

This will involve enrollment for a dedicated period of research, and there will be a minimum period of registration before you are able to submit your thesis that will form the basis of your examination. Most commonly research toward an MD ranges from 1 to 2 years, and you will need to check with the university you are planning to register with about current regulations, since these do vary and are subject to changes from time to time. There is also variability as to how these are examined – some universities will not require you to have a viva, but others make the viva a mandatory part of the exam, so this is another aspect that you will have to check locally.

In order to enroll for an MD, you must have a medical qualification. And in order to attain the doctorate, you will have to undertake a project in which you show an understanding of research and research methods and that by applying these you have been able to generate data and interpret it. The expectation is very similar to that of a PhD, as seen below, although the need to have demonstrated new ideas is less stringently applied to the MD than for the PhD in many institutions, and this can lead to some academic snobbery. Most people who have spent any time within the research environment understand that there is considerable crossover between the PhD and the MD in terms of standard of work – there are good and bad PhDs as well as good and bad MDs, and it is counterproductive to argue about the relative merits of one against the other.

You will see in the next section that the time commitment for a PhD is generally expected to be greater and that the timing of submission and examination is more strictly applied.

There are no absolutes, and it is impossible to guide you from this book as to which degree you should chose except to emphasize that you should discuss your project plan with your supervisor and discuss how they think you should aim to submit it. It is often possible to change your registration from one to another if you and your supervisor agree that this is appropriate.

Doctorate of Philosophy (PhD or DPhil)

This is the highest academic degree that can be conferred by a university except a DSc (Doctrate of Science) which serves a different purpose. It is awarded on the basis of a thesis. Although it can be based in either the arts or sciences, it is much more likely that as a clinician your doctorate will be in the science disciplines. Unlike an MD, in theory, the PhD pathway is open to all students, whether from a medical background or not. Examiners will expect to see work that represents a significant and substantial piece of research work. The Oxford University website summarizes it nicely by stating that examiners

> will be looking for work that is compatible with the work of a competent and diligent student after three or four years of full time study.

Therefore, it is not for those who expect to spend a couple of years in bed, or drinking coffee around a lab – or even doing locums and clinical work to help fund it. It requires a consistent degree of motivation and application in order to successfully complete it. If your supervisor is unhappy with your work, they may not let you submit a thesis. Indeed, the decision as to whether you can undertake either an MD or PhD may depend on you having secured sufficient funding to commit to a 2- or 3-year full-time project.

In years gone by, it may have been possible for people to hide under the banner of doing a PhD and spend many years within a university department without any significant output. With increasing financial pressures, many universities have sought to eradicate this and may require people to have demonstrated that they have the capability and motivation that are likely to enable them to attain a PhD, before allowing full registration. For students attempting to embark on a PhD following an undergraduate degree, the expectation may well be of at least a first or upper second-class degree. In some institutions, there may be an expectation that a subject will have already been studied to Masters level. There may be discretion available that will allow a department to register individuals who have demonstrated ability by other means – for instance, through professional progress or non-university qualifications. Fortunately, the basic medical degree remains unclassified (i.e., not graded) and currently meets university requirements.

It is increasingly popular for universities to register you for a probationary period. This is really to prevent students who fancy "having a go" from registering, squandering resource, or failing to achieve their aim. The implication for a university who registers a student for a PhD who then fails to complete is more than a loss of credibility – all of these facts and figures are registered and displayed by universities. More painfully for a university or department is that there is a direct financial penalty for any individual who fails to complete a PhD within the set registration time. This may vary between universities but is generally between 3 and 4 years. If you continue outside your prescribed registration time without mitigation, then they have right to charge you continuation fees. This is likely to be painful for all parties.

In general, at the end of your probationary period, you will be required to submit a written piece of work – this varies from an extended report to a mini thesis depending on the university. There may also be an oral component in the form of a *viva voce* exam in order to satisfy your department that you are ready and able to proceed and register for a PhD. The formality of this process can vary between institutions and occasionally even between different departments.

As can be seen, the commitment for both the student and the department is huge for a PhD. The penalties for failing to submit can be significant. It is tremendously rewarding to achieve this degree and should be encouraged for those whom it suits. But it is not the territory for those who are not prepared to give it their all (Table 3.1).

Table 3.1 Choosing a degree

Look at local university regulations
Talk to your supervisor about the suitability of your project
Make sure your clinical team agree to any time out
Discuss the need for prior funding

Chapter 4
Getting a Grant

With additional material from Jo Cresswell, Consultant Urologist, James Cook Hospital, Middlesbrough, UK.

For chapter summary, see Table 4.1.

Introduction

If you are a clinician entering research, you may find that you have to tolerate a reduction in pay. Established clinical academics have salaries on a par with NHS salaries; however, you may lose out on on-call supplements depending on where you work and how your contract is designed. It is important to be a little wary to whom you complain, as those pre-Ph.D. scientists working in your lab who have not come from a clinical background are often paid a lot less than you, and you will be relying on them to teach you about many aspects of your project. A little sensitivity is required to avoid causing resentment. The second point is that despite the importance of a salary to fund you as an individual, the more important aspect of research is how you will fund the project itself. It is understandable that most clinicians entering research are naïve about this, but it is worth being aware that it takes

D. Smith, D. Wood, *Research in Clinical Practice,*
DOI 10.1007/978-1-4471-2873-1_4,
© Springer-Verlag London 2013

between 9 and 12 months to get a grant, so deciding to do research a couple of months before the end of a clinical job is not realistic – at least when it comes to raising money.

There are some jobs with a set project, which have funding already secured. There are both pros and cons to this situation. The advantage may be that you are simply applying for a job, for which somebody else has (or should have) already done the planning. This avoids the headaches that will be discussed later in this chapter such as grant rejection. However, not being involved in the planning creates major disadvantages, namely:

- The ability to chose and design a project that is specific to your interests – you will simply be fitting in with the work of a department, as specified by that department.
- You will have to play catch-up in developing your understanding of the project – unless you are able to do the background reading you would have done in formulating your own project, you will use valuable time at the beginning of your time trying to cover this ground.

As to other means of funding, these are wide and varied – the advantage of a full grant is that you avoid the need for distractions. Beware of the clinical fellow job (see Chapter 2), as it is all too easy to be sucked into a job thinking that you will get time to do some research when in fact all you will do is cover service commitments for a department. This is a satisfactory option if that is what you had intended and it was clear from the outset – after all you can do some work in your own time. It becomes important and a major source of disillusionment for people to whom this is not made clear at the time of application. If you are going to achieve success in this environment, it requires a ruthless approach to time. You need to accept that this will not always be popular with colleagues. It is a common pitfall, particularly in the early stages, when research is alien and clinical work is familiar, to concentrate on the latter at the expense of the former. Inevitably, this will delay your progress in research and may lead to the failure of the project altogether.

In our field of urology, many of the happiest research fellows were those who had a grant to support their work and also managed a urology on-call commitment with an allied unit. Urology nights on call are generally relatively "low impact"; hence, they allowed the maintenance of income without interfering with their research. With the advent of MMC (Modernising Medical Careers) and hospital at night schemes, these opportunities have declined in number. Variants on this theme are those jobs that are link to a resident medical officer scheme in a private hospital. These tend to intrude more on research time as there are often bits to do at night and also involve some day work as part of a rota. However, the days are often quiet, overall, with interruptions for small tasks that can be rapidly resolved. Use this time for reading papers or grant application work, planning experiments, etc. If you subscribe to either, discuss the relative merits with your predecessor before you commit yourself.

You will need to make a judgment about the funding in your own circumstances. There is a balance between getting started as soon as possible weighed against taking on commitments that will impact on your time and therefore ability to carry out effective research. This chapter concentrates on the ideal method, that is, funding by independent grants – in our opinion, all other options are at least second best. This chapter should serve as a guide to get you started. It is not a replacement for a supervisor but it gives you an outline of when, where, and how so that when you begin to discuss these issues with your supervisor, you are familiar with the principles of the process.

Timing Your Application

The application process is lengthy and you need to factor in a 1 in 5 success rate for good projects. Each application will take you weeks to write – especially to begin with. The writing style is not the same as for a paper or abstract – it is therefore essential that you have some previous examples to read before you begin to write your own application.

The process of drafting and redrafting is tiresome but vital, and you should expect to go through several attempts before your application reaches an acceptable format. Add to this, the fact that applications are often not seen on an ad hoc basis – most grant-giving bodies will have a formal application process that requires you to submit for a deadline. Following this each application will be reviewed – in a similar way to a manuscript you submit to a journal. These reviews are then examined and a shortlist is formulated. The final selection may be made on the basis of a review of the written applications and reviewers' comments, or an interview may be offered to shortlisted applicants. If one considers the process involved in executing each part of this process (added to which some grant-giving bodies may wish to see evidence of relevant paperwork, such as ethical approval or animal licenses, each of which have their own application process), it is easy to understand that sufficient time must be allowed.

You must also make allowance for the fact that you may not be successful at the first attempt, and hence the process may extend even further. It is with all of these factors in mind that we suggest that you need to allow at least 9 months and probably a year to get a grant. You may be able to start your research before then, but if you do so it will have to be within the constraints of alternative funding.

If you are reading this with a view to starting research or you have started already and you are looking to raise grant money – begin this process today!

Where to Apply

Your supervisor will have an overall picture and experience of what has previously been successful in the area you are aiming for. Many supervisors will be actively seeking grant money all the time so may well have recommendations to make to you. This is certainly one area where initiative is allowed. You should be looking into grants and fellowships administered through your own college or specialist organizations. A number (though not all) of the colleges have formed partnerships with organizations such as the Medical Research Council or the Wellcome Foundation to provide fellowships for candidates with a project in mind. Professional organizations are increasingly following suit (if not leading the way). In the internet age, you could do a lot worse than beginning with a "Google™" (or similar) search which may throw up direct links to funding bodies or indirect pathways such as through university websites. The other search to make is for special interest groups or charities related to your area of interest since many of these organizations will run grant schemes. Some may not be huge but they may be very valuable for paying for consumables, equipment, or travel expenses – should you get the opportunity to travel to present results or learn new techniques. Do not, therefore, dismiss any grant that you could reasonably apply for. This will demonstrate to your supervisor and their department that you are committed to the project as well as providing invaluable grant writing practice. It may also provide a welcome source of money for consumables before you are able to secure longer-term, more extensive funding.

In keeping with the above, you would be wise to cast a wide net. Look at as many organizations as you can. Read the regulations that they have. Some may have specific exclusions – such as not funding work that involves animal experimentation. You are allowed to be imaginative, though not dishonest – in applying for a grant, if you feel that a different emphasis might turn a lab-based project into the search for future therapy, this may open up a whole new avenue to pursue. You also need to check the regulations regarding parallel applications. Many of the bigger organizations will not sanction simultaneous applications to other fellowships and will exclude you if you were discovered doing so. If you are thinking of trying to get away with it, there are two points of which you should be aware – the first is that as a doctor, you are bound by the conditions of good medical practice – one of which is probity. The second is grants are often reviewed by a narrow field of people – since there are only a few who are considered worthy of doing so. Those people who review for one body may well sit on the committee of another; hence, you are likely to be uncovered – it is not worth the risk as you may find that you are excluded from making any future applications.

Having said this, you may well find that once you have a fellowship, you are able to apply to other groups for small pots of additional money – such as for equipment or consumables. However, you should check with the relevant organizations first for all the reasons above. This information is readily accessible over the Internet.

On a different note, if you are aiming at achieving a grant from a large body (and some smaller groups too) such as the MRC or Wellcome Foundation, you will normally need to include some pilot data to establish the credibility of both your group and your project. This will often be clear in the application guidelines.

How to Write a Grant Application

You should not be doing this in isolation – your supervisor should be doing exactly as his or her title suggests. You should download the application form and guidelines, read them together, and firstly ensure that your project is eligible for the organization to which you are about to apply. This is a competitive process, and despite any amount of hard work put your application may nonetheless be rejected. This is important for both your psyche and the need for a contingency plan with alternative finance so your project does not falter if and when a rejection letter arrives. People often see this process in a negative light, and comments like "it is always the same people who get grants" abound in research circles. That might be true but has nothing to do with nepotism or favoritism: it is simply that good research centers write good grant applications and are therefore more likely to be successful. This goes back to some of the issues raised in Chapter 2 – no one is going to tell you where the best place to work is (everybody believes it is in their own institution); you will have to do this yourself and grant profiles (i.e., what successful grants your supervisor has) are one guide to this. As a brand-new researcher, you cannot overcome this on your own – you may be lucky, but why not stack the odds as favorably as you can – get the help of an experienced grant writer. If you have chosen wisely, your own supervisor will be ideal!

The application requirements vary enormously from a side or two of A4 with a project outline to those that require a very comprehensive form to be completed. You may find that your grant is likely to come as part of a collaborative project – in which case, you may not end up writing much of the application at all (it will be written by the heads of department or principal investigators). The most common type of application that medics complete is a fellowship. The main sections of this will be a side or two of demographics which will be straightforward and self-explanatory. There are likely to be sections about your previous jobs, awards and qualifications, publications, and career intentions. Make sure you include any prizes that you have gained as they may be important in setting you ahead from other applicants. If you have done an intercalated degree or other distinguishing work, make sure it is clearly visible as this will usually count in your favor. The inclusion of a publications section can be fairly amusing at this level. Ideally, you should have some to put in – most will not be worthy of a Nobel nomination just yet, but if you have a couple abstracts and maybe one or two other bits, then so much the better. If you are interviewed, be prepared to talk in more detail about these. Other sections will include project finance and a project outline.

Project Outline and Structure

You will be expected to give a concise outline of your hypothesis along with your proposed methodology. The structure is vital as it reflects well on you and makes it easy for reviewers to extract important information. The expected format is suggested below:

Hypothesis/Research Question
Aims/Objectives
Background
Method/Plan
Outcomes/Analysis
Timeline
Finances and Justification
References

It is helpful, in this section, to give an outline of any pilot data that you may have previously gained or that your supervisor has used to formulate the project. You should also be looking to explain how you plan to timetable the project and if possible some outline as to how the data will be handled. The basis of this is central to all projects and is something you need to discuss at the outset. In situations where you want to show a difference, for example, between two treatments, you may need to involve a statistician.

Each member of a grant committee or a reviewer has very limited time and money to give to any project put before them. Those that do not seem clearly laid out with a definite plan are much more likely to fail – no matter how brilliant the idea seems to you. It is important to read your instructions carefully – those who cannot follow instructions will not get a grant. While it is important to communicate the technical or scientific basis behind your project, do not try to blind people with science or techniques that are not widely familiar – if your reviewers cannot understand what you are getting at, they have another reason for not supporting your project.

This may all sound very negative but should emphasize that this is a highly competitive environment in which you are asking people for money to fund an unknown project in the hands of an unknown researcher. Each organization must be able to justify how they spend the money of their trustees. So you must play by the rules and make your application shine by comparison with the rest. The balance is difficult, for if your project sounds too good to be true (i.e., overambitious either in terms of the likely significance of the results or the timescale in which to achieve the work), then it probably is and once again it is less likely to gain grant money. Grant committees will also look critically at your budget and whether you can achieve your aims within it. If not, they may seek clarification or may simply reject the application on this basis alone.

Project Finance

Most grant applications require this section to be ratified by the finance department of the university submitting the application. This safeguards both the institution and the individuals by ensuring that people are quoting the correct salary scales and that your costings, including fees, consumables, etc., are realistic. You should spend some time on this as getting it wrong and underbudgeting makes life very difficult.

Many of the small grant-giving bodies will give a percentage of what you have requested with the remainder conditional on certain criteria being met. Some bodies will give you back an application and ask you to reapply if there are particular comments from reviewers that you are asked to address. Do not lose heart – keep going and do as they have requested since if they wanted to reject the application outright and give you nothing, they would have done so already. Once you have data, you can always go back and apply for additional funding. Most universities will stipulate their requirement to check an application before you submit it – you need to allow 2–4 weeks ahead of the grant deadline for this. If these are not complete (and they may take a surprising amount of time), you will be not able to submit, or you will miss the deadline and your opportunity will have been lost.

Other Issues

It is common for many organizations to ask for a lay summary, as their committees are often partly or wholly made up of lay personnel. Even those who would not consider themselves as "lay" may not be an expert in your narrow field of interest. They will rely heavily on the opinions of their reviewers, but nevertheless they will also want to understand the principles and direction of your project for themselves. It may also be useful as grant-giving bodies may use this information as means of publicizing projects that they support in order to attract additional funding for further projects. As with job applications, a good test is to find your own lay person to read it and explain your project back to you. If they cannot do this, then you need to improve your description of it!

Some committees will make their final selection on the basis of an interview. They will expect you to be able to talk knowledgably about the background of the study, your hypothesis, and your proposed techniques. You need to prepare thoroughly for this. They will understand that you are new to research, and a sensible panel will look for someone who shows promise rather than expertise. You should also be prepared for questions relating to the future clinical applications of your project.

In summary (see Table 4.1), getting a grant will make a big difference to your chances of long-term success (both in research and back in clinical practice, since getting a good grant will count in your favor with future job applications, too). Secured funding will mean that you do not have to waste time scraping money together when you could be working. The prestige attached to some grants makes attainment an achievement in its own right. Target your applications at bodies where success is more likely. Read and follow the instructions carefully. Formulate your application with a supervisor. Spend time on it and get it right and do so well before the deadline. Finally, prepare thoroughly for an interview.

Table 4.1 Getting a grant

Give yourself 9–12 months to get a grant
Apply for everything you can
Understand and follow the rules
Anticipate failure, have a contingency plan
Work with your supervisor
Keep deadlines
Prepare well for interviews

Chapter 5
Special Qualifications and Equipment

With additional material from Nikesh Thiruchelvam,
Consultant Urologist, Addenbrookes Hospital, Cambridge, UK.

For chapter summary, see Table 5.1.

In undertaking your research, as well as your aspirations to complete a dissertation or thesis, this may also be the first opportunity for you to achieve a much-coveted publication. No matter what research you are performing, most journals will require you to specify that you have acted within the proper regulatory framework relevant to your project. If the work is human, you must have appropriate ethical approval and consent in order to proceed. Many journals will turn you down flat without this in place, and you would not be the first candidate to have failed a doctorate at the viva stage because of a failure to demonstrate ethical approval. Similarly, to experiment on animals without a license or outside the license granted will result in prosecution and potential imprisonment – neither of which will look good on your CV! You will also need to maintain an up-to-date GCP (Good Clinical Practice) certificate – courses are available on line. Many universities and hospitals will also run courses on research governance and data protection.

D. Smith, D. Wood, *Research in Clinical Practice*,
DOI 10.1007/978-1-4471-2873-1_5,
© Springer-Verlag London 2013

Research and Development Registration

This is dealt with relatively easily. If you are performing any kind of clinical study within a clinical environment, you will almost certainly be required to register it with that institution's R&D committee. This is usually a straightforward process involving a short submission from you about the project – aims, methods, possible outcomes, etc. It is important to your organization as it allows a coordinated approach to work continuing under the same institutional umbrella, and it may also give you access to funding from the R&D budget.

If undertaking a clinical study involving pharmaceuticals, it is important to adhere to the Good Clinical Practice (GCP) guidelines as provided by the International Conference on Harmonisation, an international body that defines standards, which governments can rearrange into regulations for clinical trials involving human subjects. Much like the GMC's Good Medical Practice guidelines, GCP outlines standards on how clinical trials should be performed and defines the roles and responsibilities of clinical trial sponsors and clinical researchers. Many hospital R&D departments will run their own internal GCP course; if you are planning to undertake clinical trials, it would be well worth your time getting on one of these one-day courses (often free to locally employed doctors).

Ethical Approval

Like so many other things discussed in this book, this is a process rather than a one-off event. Obtaining ethical approval is therefore not something to begin on the day you start research as it may take months to be approved – if clinical research is the basis of your project, then time is too valuable to waste in this manner. You need to enquire about this in parallel with all the other vital bits of the jigsaw (grants, animal license, etc.). Failure to do so will leave you frustrated with yet another avoidable delay.

Ethical committees have an overriding responsibility to ensure that any work carried out involving patients under their auspices has a sound ethical basis, thus maintaining its duty of care to protect their interests. It is easy to dismiss this as nuisance or nonsense, but this would not be to give this important role due consideration. The committee will be made up of local and regional clinicians and other hospital staff, for example, pharmacists, nurses, laboratory staff, etc. It will also have several lay members. When you make a submission to such a committee, all have the right to read your application and raise questions of it. They are not aiming to be unreasonable, merely to carry out their responsibilities as above.

There are local ethical committees for studies involving your own institution (you can usually include two or three accessory sites) or multicenter ethical committees that are designed to deal with applications for larger studies requiring data from more centers – these are usually larger-scale pharmaceutical trials and unlikely, therefore, to be required for your own research project.

Applications are administered through the IRAS (Integrated Research Application System) - (www.myresearchproject.org.uk). This includes clear instructions and guidelines as to how to structure these – read them and follow them carefully as this will avoid your application being rejected on a technicality. You will usually be expected to include a patient information sheet and a consent form. Get hold of previously accepted examples and use these as a model. The absolute rule is to leave all jargon at the door and write in plain English. You will not be able to blind this committee with science – they are there to ensure the safety of the patients and not to referee the academic integrity of your project. They will not be impressed by terms they do not understand: if you are lucky, they will seek to gain clarification by asking you questions, but if you are unlucky, they will reject your application out of hand – they have a busy workload and simply do not have time for people who have tried to be too clever.

Once your application has been submitted, it will be circulated and read by all members of the committee. At the next meeting, they will discuss your application – you may be invited to the meeting to discuss your application. Do not be concerned about this: for some, this is routine practice, and as noted above, it may give you the chance to clarify a point that would otherwise lead to their approval being either delayed or withheld altogether. Once they have deliberated, they may suggest changes to your patient information or consent forms, and they may raise questions for you. Unless you have been invited to meet with them, you will have to answer these in writing. There are no trick questions, so keep this straightforward, and your application will work its way through as quickly as is possible.

The questions usually do not need to go before a further meeting – unless there are major doubts concerning your project. Generally, the committee will entrust the chairman to ensure the questions are answered satisfactorily and on the basis of these "chairman's action" will be taken and ethical approval be granted.

Once you have the approval, make sure that you read the small print and only do what you have been sanctioned to do – if any additional workers start on the project, you are often required to notify the ethical committee. You may also be asked to submit a progress report to the committee – failure to do so may lead to withdrawal of approval.

Licensing for Animal Research

The Beginning

Regulation to protect animals began in the seventeenth century. The current legislation is represented by the Animals (Scientific Procedures) Act 1986 which currently regulates all procedures performed on protected animals; it aims to ensure that any research using animals is original and justified. It defines protected animals as any living vertebrate (other than man!) and includes fetal, larval, and embryonic forms, and a regulated procedure is one performed for scientific purposes, on a protected animal, that has the potential to cause pain, suffering, or distress.

The Basics

The Animals (Scientific Procedures) Act 1986 is administered by the Secretary of State at the Home Office: she delegates her responsibilities to a network of Home Office inspectors who visit (sometimes unexpectedly and at random) and report upon research establishments and review license applications. Furthermore, the Secretary of State receives advice regarding license applications from the Animal Procedures Committee who annually issues a report, among other topics, on ethical processes, licensee training, and infringement details.

Any institution undertaking this work must have a Certificate of Designation which specifies a named animal care and welfare officer (senior animal technician) and a named veterinary surgeon. Responsibility for compliance with the certificate rests with the certificate holder in the institution.

Scientific procedures performed on animals must be authorized by a project license (PPL) – usually held by a supervisor and a personal license (PIL) – the focus of this chapter. Application and granting of a license adheres to the essential three R's guiding animal experimentation – replacement, reduction and refinement. Introduced in 1959, the three R's aim to find possible alternatives to animal research and potential suffering – replacement refers to the use of in vitro experiments or mathematical models to answer the scientific question, reduction refers to using fewer animals (e.g., by collaboration with colleagues), and refinement refers to altering your experimental design to minimize potential distress to animals. All experiments must adhere to these principles and any program of work involving the use of protected animals has to be justified (i.e., potential benefits must outweigh the possibility of animal suffering).

The PIL holder carries primary responsibility for the welfare of animals on which procedures have been performed. The most important aspect of obtaining a PIL is timing. As time spent in research is likely to be between 1 and 2 years in a clinical trainee's career, planning ahead is absolutely essential. It can take from 2 to 6 months to gain a PIL, so begin well in advance if this necessary to your work.

There must be a PPL within your institution before you can apply for a PIL. Once granted, the PIL is for life (subject to review), but you can only perform work within the confines of the PPL and in a venue with a Certificate of Designation. As you move jobs and projects, you can amend your personal license to include new project licenses and designated centers.

Mandatory Training Courses

To apply for a personal license, you must attend a mandatory course entitled "The Animals (Scientific Procedures) Act 1986 Training Course for Animal Users." The institution you are about to work for should be able to direct you to an appropriate venue and advise you on which modules you need to complete – once you have done this course, you can then apply for the PIL.

The Personal License Form

The PIL application form can be downloaded from the Home Office website (http://scienceandresearch.homeoffice. gov.uk/animal-research/application-forms/) along with various PIL guidance notes. The PIL application form itself has 18 sections (of which section 15 is expandable – it is important to detail all procedures you will be undertaking in this section) and is relatively straightforward to complete. In addition to the institute's PPL and the training courses, you will also need a supervisor to sign the form. The supervisor must also hold a PIL himself or herself, but does not necessarily have to be the project license holder. The purpose of supervision is to ensure the competence and reliability of the new personal licensee and to protect the animals being used.

Supervision usually remains in force for a year, and when the supervisor is happy with the licensee's technical proficiency (together with the Home Office inspector), he may then reduce the level of supervision or ask the Secretary of State to lift the supervision condition altogether. However, it is important to realize that the imposition of a supervisor does not lessen the licensee's responsibilities to comply with the Act. Take time to get this right first time – amendments are possible but time consuming.

Recent Developments

In April 1999, a new level of regulation was introduced whereby a requirement was made that all establishments have a local ethical review process to review license applications and ongoing work in addition to promoting animal welfare. This is to complement the Home Office inspectorate and not replace it. In most other countries, animal research is regulated by local ethical committee or by central government. The UK is the only country in the world that operates under both systems. Although admired for its strict controls under which animal research is conducted, the red tape surrounding license applications risks driving medical research out of the UK to countries where the welfare of animals in laboratories is not so well protected. This could easily delay (if not entirely scupper) plans for your research project. In response to this, the Expert Group on Efficient Regulation has been formed (including Home Office members), and it is envisaged that the process will remain under review and may be simplified as part of this.

Equipment

When you begin to plan your project, you will need to get a clear idea about what equipment and facilities you will need. This does not necessarily mean a long shopping list – be assured that your grant will not offer you so much money that you can completely reequip the lab! You need to start by asking what you already have, whether it works, and ensure that somebody knows how to use it and that they will be prepared to teach you. If you do not have it in your lab, there are often other labs or facilities nearby – is there available time for you to use their equipment? These are simple commonsense approaches that may avoid the need for massive capital investment or even worse buying the wrong thing.

Having made these enquiries and decided that you must have a new bit of kit, you need to thoroughly investigate the options. Look through the relevant equipment catalogues and the Internet. Talk to some companies and ask them to put you in touch with units who have the kit and arrange to go for a demonstration. It would be wise to invite your supervisor to come with you since they will keep the equipment in the lab for a number of years after you have moved on, so it makes sense for them to have close involvement.

If you are buying equipment, you may find that it is not possible to build it into your original project grant application. It is worth searching to try to find separate grants that will allow you to cover the cost of this purchase, including industry sponsors, hospital trustees, or charitable organizations. Funding may not be available through any other means, so it is important to anticipate this and be proactive.

Finally, if the equipment is of significant size or has specific requirements for function or health and safety, check with your supplier that delivery is possible – particularly if your lab is difficult to access, for example, due to a spiral staircase or absence of a lift! I have experienced delivery men who arrive with an incubator (the lab having been visited by the company reps) and refusing to carry it down four steps into the lab or suggesting that an additional charge should be paid for this – since the funding is tight, this may even be a deal-breaker (unless you pay it yourself...) and is clearly best avoided!

Summary

In many ways, this chapter will divide the readership – for some, all will apply, but for others, none will be relevant. It is vital that you add these points to your checklist early on and make enquiries. If you have not already learned it, research will teach you that unless you do something yourself, it will not happen. You cannot expect other people to spoon-feed you anymore – they all have plenty of their own things to worry about. However, if you ask people for help or how they have solved problems in the past, they will often be helpful in directing you or helping you to solve your problem.

One aspect that is the making of many but the undoing of a few, is that you have absolute ownership of a project. This makes you totally responsible for its day-to-day running and ultimately its overall outcome. This responsibility begins from the first time you take it on and means that you have to try to think of all aspects. Of course, you are unlikely to achieve this in practice, and some things you will just have to learn by experience. As one of the principal aims of this book, we hope that you will be able to avoid some of the major delays and pitfalls which are the most easily predictable.

One of the difficulties clinicians have in transferring to research is moving out of a team approach to being the sole person responsible for a project. There should always be people available to provide support, but they will not be reviewing and checking your work in the same way that happens in the clinical world. Therefore, if you forget something or do not know of its importance, then it may already be too late by the time it surfaces as a problem. Keep asking questions, learn from those around you, and if you think something might be a problem, you are probably right, so do not ignore it, but find out about it and try to correct it early on, as this will save you considerable work (and stress) in the long run (Table 5.1).

Table 5.1 Special qualifications and equipment

Consider any specific requirements you have for your project at the outset
Prepare for, and obtain these as early as possible to avoid delays when you project is in mid flow
Ethical approval is the immediate priority for any research involving patients
Identify the need for any special equipment and how you will pay for it and learn to use it
Start an application today if you will need a license for animal research

Suggested Further Reading

1. Wolfensohn S, Lloyd M. Handbook of laboratory animal management and welfare. 2nd ed. Oxford: Oxford University Press; 1998.
2. Statistics of scientific procedures on living animals. London: The Home Office Stationary Office; 2001. Command manuscript 5244 (published annually).
3. Directory of animal research training courses 2001/2002. Tamworth: Compiled and edited by the Laboratory Animal Science Association: 2001.

Useful Websites

www.ich.org The official website of the International Conference on Harmonisation explains all things GCP. Also see http://www.dh.gov. uk/en/Publicationsandstatistics/Publications/ PublicationsPolicyAndGuidance/DH_4082934 for Department of Health's UK guidance.

http://scienceandresearch.homeoffice.gov.uk/ The Home Office website and has useful information on the Animal (Scientific Procedures) Act 1986 and downloadable license application form.

www.lasa.co.uk is the website of the Laboratory Animal Science Association and lists good practice guidelines for PIL holders.

http://www.understandinganimalresearch.org.uk/ The official web-site of Understanding Animal Research, an organization founded at the end of 2008 by bringing together two UK organizations, Research Defence Society ("understanding animal research in medicine") and Coalition for Medical Progress. Details similar information as the Home Office website but in a more digestible fashion.

Chapter 6
Getting Started

For chapter summary see Table 6.1.

You may be tired of hearing that the main objective of your research is your thesis and publications, but that above all, achieving this will require focus and hard work. You do not want to be dealing with money or other worries in the meantime. You will have plenty to keep you going!

The First Day

It is not uncommon for doctors to turn up in their first day of research at the time of their usual morning ward round and expect to start making progress immediately. Our mentality is very directed and many of us expect to have recorded the first set of decent results before we go home that night. Prepare for your first disappointment! It is likely to be weeks before you are capable of running experiments correctly to produce results and months before you get anything meaningful. However, there is nothing wrong with turning up early: in fact, we think the majority of clinicians work much better by sticking to their usual routine rather than allowing themselves to slip into a more easygoing attitude of scientists and laboratory staff. Remember that, as with all your jobs until

D. Smith, D. Wood, *Research in Clinical Practice,*
DOI 10.1007/978-1-4471-2873-1_6,
© Springer-Verlag London 2013

you become a consultant, you are a visitor and you are going to have to adjust to your lab/research team's way of doing things rather than imposing your own ideas on them. Your contributions and ideas may be very valuable and some may be adopted with time, but you will have to make your way slowly – remember, a lot of people will be trying hard to accommodate you. So the first day will often be about the usual paperwork and administration. It would be good to spend a little time looking at your equipment. Why not start by reading the instruction book? You will also have plenty of background reading to do – so for idle moments, you should be able to find work to keep you occupied. Indeed, one of the important general lessons of research is to learn to use time well. You should also take the time to introduce yourself to as many people in the lab as you can. Make sure that they know who you are. Try to chat to your supervisor and arrange regular time slots for update meetings. Go and meet the administration staff who may have paperwork for you to complete – if you do not go and see them, it could take them weeks to find you! If you have not formulated a timetable for the first 6 months why not do so now – this structure will help you.

Must Have...

There are some things that will be obvious to you and one or two others that you may not have considered. Most people pay into the NHS pension scheme, and at the time of writing, this remains a good option. If you suspend payments even for a short time, you may lose some of your benefits which will take time to reaccumulate. You should take up-to-date advice (e.g., from the BMA or a financial advisor) about your contributions and what you will lose if you do not maintain these during your research. You may well find that it is sensible to continue them, with the longer term in mind, even if it means some financial hardship during your research time. Maintaining pension contributions is a straightforward process that will be organized through your payroll department – you will need to get your hands on the correct forms, complete them, and thereafter it should happen automatically – although you should check that this is the case.

It is also very important that you maintain your links with the NHS. If you are undertaking a clinical project, this will happen automatically, but if your work is laboratory based, you will help yourself by negotiating an honorary NHS contract. This is essential if you wish to collect samples for human tissue experiments or you need to question patients on the ward. This will also maintain your continuous service which will help you should you ever need to claim sickness payments or maternity leave. These may not seem like major considerations when you start research, but they will become so if either of these scenarios ever applies to you.

Locum work can seem like an attractive option to boost your income. There are a few considerations. Firstly locum work can be a fairly lonely experience, often you will not know the department or its staff and you may be expected to pick up most of the work others do not really want to do. However, it is a way of keeping your hand in and it is usually well paid. You should check your grant conditions – some will stipulate that you should not take on such work and if you are found out you run the risk of jeopardizing your funding and possibly your project. It is clearly not worth it under these circumstances. Another extremely important consideration is the day-to-day running of your project. If you are taking on locums to cover night shifts, you will not be at work the next day, and even if you are there physically, you will not be undertaking your best work. Your supervisor will detect this, sooner or later, and you may find that you alienate a considerable amount of your support network by behaving like this. You therefore need to think very carefully before you take on locum work, and if you must, chose the right time and place to do it and aim to minimize the impact on your research work.

If you do decide to do locum work, then you need to give your defense organization a ring. You may find that your level of cover will need to be increased. No one ever wants to think about making that phone call to a defense organization, but if you do have to, it is best to know that you are appropriately covered.

Starting Work

However you structure your working day, try to organize your hard copy record of your research in such a way that it mirrors the desktop on your computer. So, if you tend to organize things by time and date, then run this system throughout – then you stand a fighting chance of being able to consistently find what you seek, and quickly. One tip is to buy some A4 envelope files, and if you have a plan to cover three subject areas, you have three files, one labeled with each so that you can just drop useful bits and pieces in there – you can always reorganize them later, but until you have, you should still be able to lay your hands on what you need. Alternatively, you can use your hard-backed lab book and stick everything in there so that you can refer back to it in that way. The same is true for the potential chapters of your thesis: have a file for introduction, methods, results, and discussion. Once again this gives you a safe place to store your records – you can organize them more formally later on. Of course, to some, the prospect of organizing anything on paper is antiquated. However, the same principles apply when you are sent or you download something – create a file that allows you to find it easily. This kind of basic organization will make a big difference to you in the long run.

Write It Down!

It is good advice to write everything down from the moment you start. Times, dates, ages of patients or animals – any demographics you can lay your hands on. In your equipment file, record manufacturer details, part numbers, settings, flow rates of perfusate, and every other detail you can imagine.

In order to understand your equipment, make yourself draw a functional diagram of the setup and label it, describing the function of each part. Having collected and documented all of this information, it does not matter if the experiment subsequently goes wrong – in fact this is vital to the process of refining your methods until they work consistently. If you correct misunderstandings early on, this will make a huge difference to how easily your project moves forward and dramatically reduces the problems you will encounter with later work and when writing up. The other thing to do is that if there are particular settings that are required for the rig before you begin – you should take a digital photo of the setup. This means that when somebody else comes along and changes all the settings for a different experiment, you will be able to reset everything as you need it. You may read this section and think this is either obsessive compulsive behavior or simply dull. Both may be true, but meticulous attention to detail described above will make life easier for you and also is likely to enhance the quality of your results. It is worth giving these ideas a try – research involves constant questioning and improving of your techniques; you may develop a better system, and when you do, share it.

Without wishing to labor the point – write down EVERYTHING! It is no good trying to write up how you made a solution 2 weeks after you did it – you can easily look at the protocol and work out how you were supposed to do it but that may not be the same thing – you need to record what you actually did and how. At times you will get strange results, and understanding how these arise requires careful analysis of all data available. We had one experience where three of us were experimenting in the lab on living tissue and all sharing the same perfusing solution. Without going into unnecessary detail, calcium was an essential component of this perfusate, and in making up a new batch, one of our colleagues had become distracted and forgotten to add this. Fortunately, we were all discussing our experiments and realized that they had stopped working at about the same time.

We realized the error and were able to make up a new solution and the problem resolved. This example illustrates that with the best intentions and considerable experience, it can be very easy to make a silly mistake. At some time or other, you will over- or underdilute a reagent or omit something altogether – it is inevitable and your strange results may spoil your data. If you find you have made a mistake, then you should exclude this data from your analyses. If you find that everything was as it should be, then you should include the data – it may make the whole picture more interesting – never discard any data!

Your Working Day

You need to set yourself a realistic timetable – both for your project overall and for each day. Aim to avoid the extremes. If you are in every day of the week from 7 a.m. until 10 p.m., then you are probably doing it wrong. Similarly, if you are arriving in time for lunch and leaving in time to watch afternoon television, it is difficult to see how you will achieve anything meaningful. You need to plan ahead far more than you would in a clinical job – both on an hour-by-hour basis (for instance, if it takes 16 h to run a gel electrophoresis, this is better started at 4 p.m. One day so that it is ready for you at 8 a.m. the next day, as opposed to starting it at 8 a.m. and needing to break into the lab to rescue it at midnight!). This is also true for week-by-week plans – if you are going away on a conference, do not set up cell cultures that will need harvesting while you are away. Depending on the work you are doing, there may be times when you are waiting for tissue and then experiments run on and into the night – in some cases this is the only way to manage. If that is the case, it is sensible to let your team know and arrange to arrive later the next day – circumstances allowing.

It is acceptable to spend the odd day at home either reading or analyzing data but this should be a rare exception and certainly not the rule. Although it has become easier and easier to do this with improvements in Internet technology, you need to maintain regular contact with your supervisor and lab throughout your time with them – the majority of this must be in person. As the end of your research approaches, the time you need to spend in the lab should reduce – especially at the time you begin to concentrate on writing up your thesis. Management of this time is very individual, but most people tend to come into the lab itself on a weekly basis (more if necessary) but spend the rest of the time writing. You can only contemplate this kind of distance working once you have completed your dataset.

Expect Failures

Do not expect to turn up and have everything work for you from day one. Bits of kit will break, old bits of kit will fail – and it will take time to replace them. Cells will die when they should not; patients will decide they do not want to be involved. You will make mistakes – in fact, by the end of your project, you will probably have experienced just about everything that can go wrong!

These things will also happen to you – if you do not suffer frustration and disappointment, then you are probably not doing enough! Research is often difficult – sometimes extremely so. Remember that you are trying to discover something new – if that was easy, everybody would be doing it. Part of your research experience is learning to deal with this – stop the experiments, go back to your lab book, and analyze where things could have failed. This may be as simple as remaking a solution or replacing faulty equipment, but it may mean you need to come up with a new approach to a problem. It is always healthy to discuss your approach to a situation and to question why you are doing a particular thing – do not take it personally if someone questions what you are doing and why. Remember that amidst all this adversity, there is a real, heartfelt sense of triumph when the results start to come in and experiments begin to work.

Clinical Projects

You may find that much of the above applies whether working in a lab or on a clinical project. However, it is worth including a few words about clinical projects specifically. Clearly, ethical and trust research and development approval MUST be in place BEFORE you begin. Your team structure may be different and you need to work with them. If you are relying on other clinicians to give you data or pass patients on to you, make sure you have a strong presence. Organize to talk at departmental meetings and make time to meet people individually. Make a big effort to introduce yourself to ward, outpatient, and theatre staff as you need. Make sure you have a defined area to work in; this needs careful thought, and if you have not planned this, allocation of rooms or space may be very difficult – you and your supervisor will need strong management support to secure this. It is implicit in much of what has already been said but make sure you comply with Information Governance policies when handling any patient data.

Summary

Organization is the key (see Table 6.1). You need to come up with a system and try to stick to it. Make sure you note down everything – this may seem like a terrible chore, but it will take you 2 minutes at the time but much more to find out what you did not record when you are writing up two or 3 years down the line. Set yourself a regular timetable and keep to it. Ensure that you spend plenty of time in the lab – you will learn a lot just by being around the people who will teach you. Go to the library and read around your subject – look for new papers.

Learn to deal with the fact that you will struggle on occasions. Sometimes people have a few weeks when everything works right from the start – if you are lucky enough to enjoy this honeymoon be prepared for a fall – it will come! By planning, persistence, and regular review of your direction, you will come through it and things will begin to work well again.

Table 6.1 Getting started

Write everything down
Stick to a timetable
Create a system for collecting information
Expect mistakes and failures
If things fail look at why
Take advice and help if you need it

Chapter 7
Data Management

For chapter summary see Table 7.1.

Data that emerge during your productive period of research will be the foundation stone that underpins the rest of your work. When you come to publish your work or be examined upon it, this will be the most closely interrogated part of any discussion that arises. It is therefore imperative that you learn how to produce good data, how to process and analyze that data, and then how to present it. The aim of this chapter is to give you a guideline on which to build. There are so many different forms of data that it would be impossible to give an in-depth discussion without monopolizing the whole book.

Unfortunately, some people progress through research without ever understanding the importance of their data. Those theses that consist of thick slices of introduction and discussion on either side of wafer-thin results and methods section are likely to be more critically examined at the time of the viva.

D. Smith, D. Wood, *Research in Clinical Practice,*
DOI 10.1007/978-1-4471-2873-1_7,
© Springer-Verlag London 2013

Getting Started

When you begin any experiment, you may need to calibrate your equipment. You must do this yourself. If anyone offers you calibration data, by all means use it for a couple of dry runs but then get your own and keep it on file. It is reasonable to be asked about your calibration at any time during your work, and you need to have a full understanding of it. This can only really be achieved on the basis of personal, practical experience.

Early Data

It is truly exciting when you begin to produce your first results. This is why you have entered research – to find answers – and those answers will come from your data. Just like learning to clerk a patient, it takes a huge amount of practice before you begin to produce reliable data. It is an additional skill to be able to undertake the appropriate analysis and then to present it in a manageable form.

Do not be disappointed if you find, as you progress, that your early data look wildly different from the results you get later. It probably means that your technique is improving and your data are becoming more reliable. This is part of "method development" that you may wish to discuss in your thesis – particularly if there are changes that you made to your methods on the basis of personal experience that helped to improve the consistency of your results.

The majority of people end up disregarding the data they accrue within their first 6 months. It is often inconsistent and therefore unreliable, having been collected during a time that you were developing and refining methods and hence not useful in building your final argument. However, you should still keep a careful record of all these early data so that you can refer back at any time. It may be that it is more useful than you expect – especially when you come to write up your results. You are likely to feel that this early time when results are not coming is time that is being wasted. It is not. This is vital time during which you develop an expertise in the technical elements of your project, as well as develop your understanding of the scientific method. However, it is easy to become frustrated with your apparent lack of progress and lose motivation. Use this time to write some of your introduction. This will help to give you a sense of achievement, otherwise lacking in your day – you may also encounter a paper describing a different approach that helps to solve your problem.

You need to develop a system, early on, that allows you to cross-reference any analyzed data with raw traces or data collection sheets and lab book entries. This may be important as it is easy to make mistakes, and when you find inconsistencies, it is then much easier to retrace your steps and look for how the problem arose. Some people invest in high-powered statistics packages that allow data to be fed in and have it returned in any form required. The clear advantage to this is that it is quick and within reason will help you find that answer you want. However this approach has something of a "black box" mentality – unless you can explain why you analyzed data in a particular way and the steps you took in doing that, you will not fully understand your data and your final interpretation may suffer as a result. You have to be an expert on your own data – you, and hopefully your supervisor, are the only people who will be. Therefore, it is vital that you understand the process that has led to your answer. It is not good enough simply to have an answer that appears to fit.

Building Data

When you first start to process and analyze your data, you must keep a copy of the raw data on file and maintain this practice throughout. This means that if you make a mistake in analyzing it that you cannot unravel, you can at least go back to the start and the original data is not lost. It is also vital that you have your data backed up. It is worth backing it up in at least three places, such as burning onto CD or USB stick and a copy on your supervisor's computer – as well as on your own laptop. The loss of your data would be devastating and you will meet people that have experienced this – do not let it be you. It is essential that you comply with the Data Protection Act and the local policy for implementing this. The principle behind this is that no patient-identifiable data should be transported outside a trust and that any data that is stored should be deleted once no longer required.

If you follow these simple rules you then have the flexibility to do whatever you like in analyzing your data. You can really explore the possibilities and analyze it in multiple ways. This may sound slightly strange, but it means that you learn a number of things. Not only will you find the real answers about your data but you will learn a variety of methods for looking at data, how they work, when they are useful, and what happens to data when certain tests are applied. This may end up being totally irrelevant to your current research, but it may be invaluable to you in the future when you come to write another project up, as well as for your ability to critique the literature.

Remember, your time in research is not just about producing results and writing a thesis. You should be aiming to develop a number of skills as part of this, and data interpretation should be one of them.

It is useful to sit down with people who have had experience of data handling – ideally in your own area – as they will start to give you an impression of what to look for and how to move forward. Learning these skills may save you a lot of time in the future. This kind of advice will also lead you to the correct analysis of your data. Depending on the size and complexity of your project, you may need to use the services of a statistician at regular intervals. There is no shame in this, but you must be open about it in your thesis discussion, as you will feel very exposed in a thesis viva if you are asked to give detailed explanations about analyses that you do not fully understand.

Keeping Track

It is very easy to get to the end of a day or week of experimenting and file your raw traces or data in a folder to sort out at a later date. In some ways, this may even seem an attractive option. However, what your data shows you as you go along may be vital to the overall success of your project. Therefore, it is sensible to analyze your data on a regular basis. This means processing all your raw data, using appropriate statistics, and plotting the data graphically. This will tell you a number of things, but most importantly it will tell you when you have done enough of the correct experiment to have meaningful data. It will tell you if the experiment is working and, if not, allow you to rethink and reconfigure it. In rare cases, it may even tell you that you need to consider a complete change of direction. It is vital that you keep up with regular analysis of your data. When you are in full swing with your project, data will come in rapidly in particular chunks of productivity – in general, 6–8 months of meaningful data collection is likely to provide sufficient good data on which to structure your thesis.

Writing Up

When you collate your final results, you must check that you have been consistent with your analysis. Over the course of 2 or 3 years, your thoughts may have changed, even if only subtly, and this may make a difference to your overall interpretation.

The data that you base your conclusions on will clearly be your most consistent data, but as said above, it may be useful to show some early data to justify your reasons for a change in methods. It is also useful to show examples of your raw data so that anybody reading your record can see how you got from one stage to the next and so on.

Divide your data into clear parts so that you can discuss it in manageable sections. This will make it easier for you to think and write clearly about it, and your reader will benefit

Table 7.1 Data management

Keep all data
Organize data and cross-reference it
Analyze it at regular intervals
Analyze it yourself
If you need help to analyze it – be open about it
Think about how you want to present it
Divide data into manageable sections

in the same way. You can draw it all together as part of your discussion with reference to previous work but your own thought processes must be clear.

In summary, data are the cornerstone of your work, and when you begin to obtain real data, they will create a genuine excitement. You should, with time, get better at obtaining data – this shows an improvement in both your skill and understanding. All data that you obtain should be kept in its raw form – even if you think it is so bad that you may not use it in your final presentation. You should try to analyze it as you go along as this will help to tell you if you have enough data and if there are any problems with your method. It also allows you to divide data into manageable chunks – this will further help you when you are writing up your work and also those who need to understand it (Table 7.1).

Chapter 8
Writing Up

For chapter summary, see Table 8.1.

If you successfully complete your thesis, you will automatically put yourself in the top 50 % of people who undertake research. It is a hidden disgrace that so many people fail to convert 2 or 3 years of research into written form. Not everyone is aiming for a thesis but most begin with that objective. There are computer hard drives the world over littered with incomplete work – do not let yours be one of them!

Writing up will take longer than you ever imagined, cause you more upset, stress, and frustration than you ever thought possible, and will significantly impact on your social and family life. It is often set aside as though there is an assumption that it will be easy and therefore will "just happen." In fact, second only to the early disappointments of experimental and method development, this is often one of the most frustrating and difficult times in your research. It is also one of the few tangible things that you can be judged by at the end of your research project – hence, there is good reason to get it right.

It is sensible to consider why writing up is such a difficult process. Your principle aims in producing a thesis are twofold: firstly to give a reasoned account of your work in order to

D. Smith, D. Wood, *Research in Clinical Practice*,
DOI 10.1007/978-1-4471-2873-1_8,
© Springer-Verlag London 2013

demonstrate your findings and provide a foundation for your conclusions – clearly with a view to your higher degree. The second is to produce a document that would allow a reasonably intelligent adult to duplicate your work. That person may even be you wishing to resume the project after a time delay – this is an important principle. Putting together an experiment to try and prove a hypothesis can be extraordinarily frustrating. There will be regular failures and difficulties, some of which may be insoluble and lead to a complete change of direction. With persistence, development of your own expertise, and some luck, the experimental protocol starts to fall into place and you manage to produce some meaningful data for your thesis. The most fruitful period of data collection in a 3-year project may be as short as 6 months. Your early data may be unusable apart from as an illustration of your method development. The period in your project when things are working and the data is rolling in is your delayed honeymoon. If you have gone into research in the right frame of mind, it will be one of the most fulfilling times of your life. You will have invested an enormous amount of time and effort to reach that point and, finally, you have arrived! During this time, you will feel good about yourself and hopefully, your supervisor will reinforce this by agreeing with how good your data is. This is the time in which you are establishing new evidence. Towards the end of this period, the reality of the next stage needs to hit home – writing up. It is easy for it to not to and for you to make the mistake of many and carry on doing experiments that you enjoy seeing bring in yet more apparently valuable data. This is an understandable error but nevertheless a foolish one. If you have sufficient data, set a date and stop experimenting. To carry on creates added difficulties in the long run since you will have more data to analyze and less time in which to do so before returning to clinical practice. To write up takes a variable amount of time – depending on you, your supervisor, and your project. For most, it is around 6 months, some have done it in less and for many, particularly if it extends beyond your time in research into your next jobs, it is a form of prolonged torture.

In order to write up effectively, you will need to withdraw from the lab environment. The most successful people who wrote up within a set time frame were able to motivate themselves to do so from home or library but definitely outside the laboratory where there are many distractions – including the temptation to do "just one more" experiment. That said, you need to maintain regular, face to face contact with your supervisor. Your time management during this phase must be ruthless – you should avoid presentations and going to meetings as these are distractions that will hinder your progress. It can take a couple of months to appreciate this but once grasped, it makes a big difference.

In any event, wherever you do the actual writing, the process itself is no more or less painful. Suddenly, the praise that you were receiving for producing good data turns to an eternal nagging for the next chunk of thesis and then disdain when you deliver as this means MORE reading for your supervisor. Remember, this is hard work for both of you.

The "How to" Guide of Writing Up

This is an intensely personal experience. You will probably never spend such a long period of time alone, even when working for exams. The biggest advantage you can gain is to start from the beginning with your lab book. In this, you should have recorded and drawn/photographed everything (dial settings, brands, batch numbers, amounts, changes, thoughts, etc.) no matter how dull it seemed at the time. The less you record at the time, the greater the chance that you will have to spend hours going back to the laboratory to gather this essential information. It can be done but it is a huge waste of time to do so at this stage of the project. Furthermore, since your "time out" writing up, some pieces of equipment may have been moved, or worse still replaced, making obtaining the details more difficult. The second is to use the advantages of the computer age. Spare a thought for senior staff who can recount their tales of handwritten thesis being given to secretaries to type and then having to deal with their corrections. In the age of the computer and user-friendly word processing packages, it does not matter what you write to start with, as you can change it – literally – at the touch of a button. Therefore, when you do an experiment, write your method up on your computer after you have done it. Ideally, record all the mundane data that we have already suggested above (see Chapter 7). If you later change the method, rewrite it (but keep the original). In this way, by the time you reach the point of writing up you will have the bare bones (at least) of your materials and methods chapter. This can be reshaped and refined as many times as you like but it is a lot easier to do it this way than it seemed for those who tried to write it retrospectively.

There is a similar counsel of perfection for results chapters. If you are wise, the majority of the leg work for these can be done as you go along. Certainly, your data analysis can be remolded into formal chapters. This is slightly harder than with the materials and methods, but the aim is not to have written the whole thing to perfection before you have finished experimenting but to make the process of writing up more manageable and perhaps less painful.

It is sensible to consider in this the position of your supervisor and how (psychologically) you can tip the balance marginally in your favor. It is infinitely more achievable for any of us to sit down and read a few pages or one chapter rather than a whole book at once. If you present your supervisor with your entire first draft in bulk, the likelihood is that you will not see it for several months. It can be very difficult to get back into writing after such a delay, not least because by then you may well be back in a full-time clinical job. If you offer a chapter or section at a time, these can be read in a reasonably short time and hence you are likely to get it back for correction much more quickly. In the meantime, you can have started work on the next section. This is by far the most efficient and effective way of producing your thesis as lessons learned from the first correction can be applied to subsequent submissions – hence, they should take up less of your supervisor's time as you write more.

In terms of order, there are many different viewpoints. There seems to be logic to writing your methods first since this gives you the experimental nuts and bolts of your project. It also requires relatively little grasp of the background literature – at least to write a draft – and you can plug any holes later. It is, quite simply, an account of what you have done.

The second section to tackle is the results. These are your outcomes and all your discussion will revolve around these so it is as well to thoroughly understand these next.

Your discussion will allow you a final close inspection of your results as compared with the relevant literature and the chance to develop themes from your own thinking about the way your research has gone. This may be very different from your original project plan – look back at your grant proposals to review this. While *you* may consider your work to be worthy of a Nobel laureate, it is important to have discussed your views with those around you to keep your feet more firmly on the ground and avoid making grandiose statements in your conclusions. Finally, albeit paradoxically, comes your introduction – although you may have written sections of it to keep busy in your early days. If so, you can accept, rewrite, or flatly reject your previous efforts. This is the part of your thesis that you want to define the background that explains the road you have taken and to set the scene for your reader to understand and appreciate the contribution that your work has made to the field. By the time a reader has finished your introduction, they should be calling for some experiments to be done and if you have written it well, they will be the very same experiments that you will go on to describe in your methods and results. It is much easier to achieve this if you finalize the introduction at the end of the writing process rather than the beginning.

That said, part or all of any section can be written at any time and subsequently altered if needs be. It is sometimes helpful to write down important quotes or views from the literature that form a foundation for your work.

The introduction also contains the background to your work – hence, as suggested in Chapter 7, you may begin to write some of it in the early stages of your project as it will help to build familiarity with your subject and may help solve some early problems. It is sensible to record your thoughts at the same time. Any or all of this may change with time – but at least you have a starting point. Keep everything in an ordered fashion so that you can find it again. Develop a system of filing, as suggested in previous chapters, so that throughout your project if you get a reference or piece of information that you think might be useful, you have got a safe place to put it and review it when the time comes. This is a vital and time-saving requirement that you will come to appreciate later on.

It is sad to have to mention plagiarism, but when reading a thesis or essay, it is surprisingly easy to pick up on a variation in writing styles. Many universities will have very strict rules on plagiarism and may require you to vet your submission by running it through a system that looks for similarities. The bottom line is do not steal other peoples' ideas but acknowledge their work and give due credit. This should still allow ample opportunity for your own work, thoughts, and ideas to stand out.

Reference Managing Software

Just a short comment on these. Some people swear by them but others have never had great success, probably due to a lack of persistence. The alternative is to cut and paste things around which is all very well until you decide you need to change everything or even just need to add a reference on the first page of your introduction! Some of the modern packages will alter your reference list accordingly, which saves a lot of time. The most up to date will use an online system such as Mendeley which allows formation of groups – this may be useful for you and your supervisor and later for others to contribute to peer-reviewed publications. The best advice is to try one or two out and see how you get on. If it works for you then use it, but if not – it is not the end of the world.

Publications

There is no universal advice about this. There are many articles that offer suggestions and advice on how to get things published. The most sensible method is to write your first few papers with someone who is already well published. This will help you to avoid some of the pitfalls. With this experience on board, you can then reread your literature on how to get published and it will all fall into place. You will develop your own style and one of the frustrations is that senior authors have also done this and each is slightly different. Having just understood how one person works, you may well be moving on to the next who has a different style and will want different things from you. That is life and it is safer to adjust to it than to expect others to change for you. It is beyond the scope of this book to advise you on how to get your work published apart from using the above as your starting point. If your work is good and you have sensible advice, you will be successful in this. Regrettably, if you have poor data or you are badly advised, your chances of success will be reduced.

The philosophy that we adopted was that it was more important to produce a thesis than peer-reviewed publications. Once you have completed your research, there will be ample opportunities for you to write papers in the peer-reviewed literature. Whereas writing a thesis requires your own self-motivation and effort for your own reward, other people will be keen to help you with a paper as there is a degree of benefit for them. Apart from your supervisor, fewer people will be so sympathetic about your thesis – especially once you have left the laboratory. Many will venture the alternative view that a series of peer-reviewed papers will form the basis of your thesis either as separate chapters or combining the methods and results, leaving you to tie it together with a unifying discussion. You should approach in the way most suited to you, after discussion with your supervisor.

In summary (see Table 8.1), just get your thesis written! To fail in delivering this is a failure of your time in research. There are many distractions, most of which are infinitely

Table 8.1 Writing up

Write up – do not fail to do this
Break it up into sections
Use what you have already written (draft sections or previously published papers)
Keep going
Try to stay out of the lab but in contact with your supervisor

more appealing than sitting alone in a room and getting down to some writing. Avoid them, including professional meetings and the temptation to get your name in lights. There are exceptions to every rule and the authors understand the pressures of publishing ahead of others in certain circumstances. However, a completed thesis is likely to count for more than a published paper (the letters from your degree will remain after your name forever) and so our advice stands, particularly as an uncompleted thesis may count heavily against you. Set yourself time and a timetable for completion; write up in manageable sections, keep close contact with your supervisor, but keep out of the lab.

Chapter 9
An Academic Career Pathway

With contribution from Hashim Ahmed MRCS BM BCh BA(Hons), MRC Clinician Scientist, Division of Surgery and Interventional Science, University College London, UK.

For a chapter summary, see Table 9.2.

Background

Approximately 20 years ago in countries such as France and Germany, there was a reduction in academic funding with universities ceasing to invest in an academic future which has, in large part, been corrected with appropriate investment from their government. A similar concern has been developing in the UK, where, according to the Walport Report:

> Warning bells have been ringing for some time over the perilous state of academic medicine and dentistry in the UK.
> (Taken from Dr. Mark Walport's report 2005: Report of the Academic Careers Sub-Committee of MMC and the UKCRC)

D. Smith, D. Wood, *Research in Clinical Practice,*
DOI 10.1007/978-1-4471-2873-1_9,
© Springer-Verlag London 2013

This report and Sir David Cooksey's report (2006) the following year were commissioned to give recommendations for the training of researchers and educators of the future (Walport) and how this should be funded in the most effective and efficient way (Cooksey). These reports recognized a fundamental lack of structure and function to overall research in healthcare alongside a lack of clear career planning, funded posts, and systematic flexibility. There is an acknowledgment that with current process and pressures in the NHS, there is likely to be a shortfall between the expectation regarding the progress that existing staff can deliver in a research environment with what is realistically achievable in practice.

Sir David Cooksey's report tackles a number of central issues and suggests a merger of budgets with the Department of Health and the Medical Research Council. In tandem with the creation of the Office for Strategic Coordination of Health Research (OSCHR), this approach aims to provide a more cohesive and better coordinated approach to research. Another more recent report – Best Research, Best for Health (2009) suggests that an overall improvement in access to research-related funding would improve the ability of centers to achieve grant funding ("regardless of location") on the basis of merit. As a result of the ongoing investment to establish the NHS as a world leader, a health-related, research-led culture, this report also sets a clear vision of improving access for all centers, and therefore patients, to take part in clinical trials. Its overall mission "to create a health research system in which the NHS supports outstanding individuals, working in world-class facilities, conducting leading-edge research, focused on the needs of patients and the public" is reaffirmed in the National Institute for Health Research 2009 report.

An outline appreciation of the reports above serves to inform us of a growing government recognition and enthusiasm for health-related research: if ever there was a time for trainees to capitalize on such opportunities, now is the time!

Opportunities

In addition to the government recognition of the importance of high-quality research, the practicality of developing a career that includes protected academic time has never been greater. In medical schools, the development of MB-PhD programs aims to begin the process early and encourage keen academics to lay down an early marker. Academic F2 jobs allow those already working as junior doctors to spend a 4-month spell sampling and participating in research or to integrate with research throughout the year – either are valuable opportunities and the Walport report suggests piloting a link between these posts and the MB-PhD program (Table 9.1).

These represent focused opportunities for individuals to participate in, learn about, and perhaps pursue academia. This creates a far more structured environment than was previously the case and may well draw more people in to research as well as producing better outcomes for both individuals and institutions.

For those at a higher stage of medical training, the Academic Clinical Fellowships (ACFs) are year-long schemes that allow trainees to spend 25 % of their time working in research. It is a common misconception that academic clinical fellows are expected to have achieved an MD by the end of this – this is not the case. These posts are aimed at those early in their specialist training and are designed to allow those successful in gaining such a place to undertake a project, collect data, and work toward a competitively funded research project at the end of their year. Of course, the time and data already accumulated may well be included in any subsequent work toward a PhD or MD. It is expected that there will be an attrition rate between ACFs and ACLs – there are 2–3 ACF posts per ACL. This is deliberate and designed to ensure survival of the fittest – there is no room for complacency.

Clinical lectureships are aimed at those trainees with National Training Numbers (NTN) and who are completing a PhD-MD who wish to continue their academic work. These

Table 9.1 Outline of academic career path

Timing	Academic milestone	Comments
Medical school	MBBS	
	Intercalated BSc	
	MB-PhD	
Foundation program	Academic foundation posts FY1/2	Part-time clinical with academic component
Specialist training Academic clinical fellowship	During ST 1, 2, and 3 with 20 % devoted to research	Time can be used flexibly, i.e., 1 day per week or one complete week in 5
Specialist training Academic clinical lectureship	Senior trainees ST 4, 5 May combine with clinician scientist fellowship which may extend into senior lecturer or consultant role CCT expected here	ST training may also be interrupted by personal fellowship to undertake PhD or MD project – this will usually build to the ACL role
Academic position	Senior lecturer	
	Further clinical training	
	Senior clinical lectureship	

posts are for those wishing to pursue postdoctoral research, offering academic and clinical training in a 50:50 ratio. They may run throughout training up until the award of CCT but may end sooner on attainment of a national "clinician scientist" award, appointment as a senior lecturer, or the gaining of an MRC or Wellcome Trust Grant. It is possible for those who enter these schemes but find that it is not suitable for them to leave the academic training and to re-enter full-time clinical training at any point. For this reason, the posts are closely linked with NTNs, and an application for any clinical lectureship post aimed at senior trainees will be either:

- Linked with a NTN (i.e., appointed simultaneously)
- Dependant on the candidate already having a NTN

When you apply for such a post (particularly if it is for both an NTN and ACF or ACL at the same time), you must be clear about the essential criteria for the post you are aiming to obtain; otherwise, you could waste considerable time and effort applying for something for which you are not eligible. All deaneries have strictly limited numbers available, and no post, academic or otherwise, can be used as a means of gaining a training number through a "back door." Check the regulations when you come to apply – you need to be clear.

The "Old Fashioned" Way

With all of these changes, the need for conventional time out for research at whatever stage might be questioned. A more "seamless" training that is the goal of MMC may mean that some will be deemed clinically ready for consultant jobs at a younger age than has previously been possible, particularly in the surgical specialties. Some will take that opportunity as soon as it presents itself, while others may prefer to develop a subspecialty interest, or find that they cannot compete for the jobs that really interest them without doing further "fellowship" style training. The anecdotal predictions remain that for those who wish to improve their chances of gaining a subspecialty fellowship or consultant job are likely to undertake a period of research to demonstrate their commitment to that particular area of practice…. This may well be at a more senior stage than was the case in the last 10 years or so (when research was done after the SHO stage, before obtaining starting on "Calman" SpR training) but more similar to the situation of 20 years ago (when research was done between the transition from registrar to senior registrar status).

Either way, research is likely to continue to be pursued by committed individuals wishing to raise their career profile and their chances of the right consultant post. It may include two cohorts – those who obtained one of the aforementioned academic roles and those who have realized their research ambitions later in their clinical career....

There are some important points that merit emphasis:

• Academic clinical combined training should not necessarily, even in craft specialties, lead to a lengthening of CCT. There is a need to assess competencies and balance service provision such as extra clinics, endoscopy lists, and diagnostic lists. With negotiation, these can be removed from timetables to accommodate the academic sessions without detriment to clinical training – this needs to be set up before you begin and emphasizes the need for management engagement by your supervisor.

• Out of program research (e.g., MD or PhD projects) should be recognized for training prospectively via STC/Deanery/SAC/PMETB. This process takes about 6–9 months so you need to start informing everybody at an early stage.

In summary, the current era may represent a golden age for academic medicine with new opportunities and strategies for those keen to pursue research. Success can bring with it a senior academic post and HEFCE funding – this will depend on your delivering according to expectation. Whatever stage in your career you consider this, you need to carefully review and consider your options because it is increasingly true that they exist and are there for the taking (Table 9.2).

Table 9.2 An academic career pathway

The Walport and Cooksey Reports demonstrate that there is a real commitment to support excellent opportunities for academic clinical practice
An academic clinical fellowship is a good place to start working toward a period of research, gaining experience and data to stimulate getting a grant
After completion of a higher degree, an academic clinical lectureship allows post doctorate research combined with 50 % clinical practice and may lead to an increasing time in research as a clinical scientist or senior lecturer

Chapter 10
Getting Back

For a chapter summary, see Table 10.1.

Getting a Job

Getting back into a clinical post has changed significantly since we completed our research. You will have to wade through the new application process which remains a subject under review – and is likely to remain under refinement for the sometime to come. Application forms are readily available and can be downloaded from the net – you should do this well in advance to ensure that you have all of the essential and as many desirable criteria as possible – you can then fill in any gaps as soon as possible. It is clear that much more emphasis is now being placed on interpersonal skills, such that you may have to describe various scenarios and how you have influenced the outcome. These may include difficult clinical situations or other evidence that allows you to demonstrate good communication skills. Your feelings about whether this is an appropriate assessment are not relevant (at least at the time you are reading this chapter). If this is likely to form part of your application, you will have to complete the form and the process as it stands and compete along with your peers.

D. Smith, D. Wood, *Research in Clinical Practice,*
DOI 10.1007/978-1-4471-2873-1_10,
© Springer-Verlag London 2013

As the process becomes tried and tested, the strengths and weaknesses of candidates who are successful will become clearer. It is beyond the remit of this book to suggest a way through the current appointment process, but it is likely that, as with previous dramatic changes in medical career structure, the basic essentials will still apply.

Start Early

No matter which stage of your career you have reached, you need to keep thinking about where you are heading next, and this certainly applies to your plans after you finish your research. Your project should not be an isolated event but should be part of a carefully planned career structure. As we have said earlier, you should discuss your research with both academic and clinical mentors – this is not just in relation to whether everybody thinks this is a good project or not but also where it is likely to take you. It is something of an art form but when you become a research fellow, you need to work at maintaining a profile within your specialty. This should be done on a number of different levels.

You should keep your local consultants and mentors up to date with your progress and plans. You may also be able to help with one or two small clinical projects that will keep you in peoples' consciousness. As your research work goes on you need to present it regularly – in the lab, to people who have given you tissue and/or ethical approval, to your referees, and at meetings and conferences. Many people think that it will be easy to talk about their own work. To be able to stand up and speak lucidly about any subject is a skill and needs development. Talking clearly about something in which you are engrossed and expert to an audience which may be unfamiliar with your work provides a particular challenge. Any accomplished presenter who you watch today and assume they were gifted with a natural ability has worked very hard to achieve that level of polish.

You may be having a break in a rotation in order to carry out research. In which case, you will not have to apply for a new job but the above points are still relevant. If you are at a senior stage in your career, you will, almost certainly, have very specific objectives when you return to the wards. You will have realized by this stage in your career that you will need to start maneuvering for your chosen senior years on a rotation early on, and you may even be doing this with a longer term view of a particular consultant appointment. No one else will do this planning for you. It is usually sensible to lodge a request, in writing, well in advance. This will be no guarantee but it is evidence of your intention that you can produce if things become difficult later on. Your main advantage is that you will be known to the key trainers, and they can assume your ongoing interest and motivation to follow your evolving career plan. It also means that you are likely to remain within the ARCP (or previously the RITA) review process and have a designated slot to go back to – fine-tuning of that will take some effort but will be well worth it.

You will be expected to maintain your regular paperwork throughout your research time. This will include a research portfolio. Those people assessing you may expect you to be showing achievements from day one. This is an impossible situation and one which at times you may just have to ask for their understanding. Perhaps the best defense if you do not have a finished paper to show is to provide a record of your local presentations and a plan for your publications including a time line.

If you have not yet gained a place on a clinical rotation, you need to ensure that you are fully up to date with the current application process. This may take time and be cumbersome. Look at the form and the criteria well in advance. Think of it like a game. That is not intended to belittle the process but merely to emphasize that anybody and everybody will be aiming to make themselves appointable and if they can find away to gain an extra point by abseiling off Big Ben then be sure that they will do so. You have to be looking to ensure that you have *ALL* the essential criteria and *AS*

MANY of the desirables as you can. In fact if you apply logic to it, the desirable criteria are more important discriminators than the essential ones, which do not discriminate at all between short-listed candidates, who must, by definition, all possess these (see earlier discussion – Chap. 2).

If you do not have essential criteria, you cannot be considered for appointment: your application will simply go straight to the rejection bin. Remember, there are likely to be many more applications than places available and if you cannot demonstrate enough commitment to fulfill the essential criteria, how is anyone going to believe that you are worthy of such a valuable placement? If you do not have the essential criteria, then make sure you do before the next application round, and try again then. Therefore, people only start to separate themselves with desirable criteria – of which research has often been one. In years gone by, since the majority of people started to fulfill this desirable criterion, it had become virtually impossible to get a job without having done it. In a competitive market, it therefore becomes almost essential by default. However, the emphasis of research is being reevaluated in the current application process for training.

While it would be naïve to extrapolate from this that research will have no value in the revised process (the need for research training will simply reemerge at another stage), the system may well work to discourage research merely for the sake of it. However, if you plan to pursue any kind of specialist career, you will be competing against a self-selecting and highly motivated bunch, a group that needs little or no prompting when it comes to ways of increasing their competitive standing. Hence, if everybody is able to become a seamless trainee but cannot select their discipline unless they achieve a high ranking, people will find a way to achieve this. Research shows commitment and the ability for self-direction and may be used as a desirable criterion to demonstrate this. Even if it is not deemed valuable at the entry stage of specialist training, it may become so at the time of consultant appointments. Its intrinsic value will therefore remain unaltered; it is simply the timing that will change.

It is important to emphasize that, while research has traditionally been a way of gaining a competitive edge, this should never be the sole motivation for those undertaking it – the value of research runs much deeper as has been discussed previously.

The Application Process

No matter how it is dressed up, whether old fashioned or new fangled, this is a difficult process. The aim is to appropriately select people who can show an ability to learn and succeed in a demanding role. It therefore aims to detect those individuals who are most likely to make the best of these precious opportunities. You cannot begin preparations for this early enough – start to look into what you have to do, tailor your CV to be attractive for the job you are aiming for, and work hard both at what you are doing in research while maintaining a profile in clinical practice – this is difficult to do but vital for success. Specialist training jobs are not designed for people who are waiting for an opportunity to be handed out on a plate but are for those who are actively focused on achieving their chosen career.

It would be quite impossible to give you the details of how best to complete an application form, but in a similar way to the grant application process, begin by asking about other (successful) people's previous experiences. You can benefit by getting your senior colleagues (registrars and consultants) to look over your application form – if so, give them enough time to do so properly – you will benefit less if they only have time to glance through it and spot obvious spelling mistakes. It is perfectly acceptable to highlight those points that you think favor your appointment to the role for which you are applying. Never lie, however – there have been examples of candidates who have cited a number of papers they had supposedly written on application forms. When these are checked, just before interview, and found to be fictitious – it leads to a fairly uncomfortable interview and certain failure in the application process, as well as significantly tarnishing, if not outright destroying, your reputation and that of your unit. Make sure that your application is delivered in plenty of time – you should get some form of evidence that it has met the deadline, just in case of problems later on....

The Interview

Once your form is completed and submitted, you will have an anxious wait until the short-listing process is complete. When the results are available, check any information you are given (good or bad) as there are short-listing anecdotes that happen because the person giving out information (particularly if this is done by telephone rather than official letter) simply has read out the wrong details – this is extremely unpleasant and distressing.

In the interim, you can start to do some of the background reading for your interview preparation. Read the newspapers and look for relevant articles. Read the BMJ news section – this is a very good way of getting an insight into current medical politics. "Hospital Doctor" is also another excellent source of information about current medical politics. You then need to start to probe more deeply – including the various Department of Health websites relating to recent issues, the NHS websites, and any relevant articles. You need to sell yourself as a consultant of the future rather than tomorrow's registrar. This is important and demands a carefully prepared mindset. For instance, if you are asked about junior doctors' hours, it easy to say that you do not agree with the changes – that may even be how you feel. However, you need to demonstrate that you can take on the problems this might engender and adapt yourself to manage the changes to give the most positive outcome for you and those around you. This is clearly a much stronger answer: it demonstrates that not only have you understood the changes in junior doctors hours, and appreciated that it may have an impact on both training of juniors in the future and delivering a satisfactory service to patients, but have shown the positive response that with careful planning and consideration, these potential problems should be surmountable. Of course, you then have to have some ideas about how these changes might be managed but for trainee interviews, these will not need to be very detailed. The consultants appointing you do not want to hear about your day to day complaints; they want to know that if they have to sit alongside you in a few years time you are going to be a member of their (or any other) department who will contribute in a positive way. We have given a number of practice interviews with trainees and it is very clear to pick out those who have grasped this concept and those who have yet to – there is a strong correlation with those who go on to get a job.

You can expect questions on a few standard areas such as audit and clinical governance. You are likely to be asked about managing a clinical scenario and may also be asked to describe your approach to a difficult situation. It is also possible that you will be asked to talk about a paper you have read recently – so prepare one! A good question to be asked is: "what is the most clinically relevant part of the research you have done?" Again, you need to have a thought-out answer ready. With a quick internet search, you can find a number of sites that will offer you a series of sample questions – you can practice many of these among a group of friends. You may find it strange that you know many of the people you are applying against – this only gets worse as you get further up the tree. Get used to it, prepare well, and accept between you that there will be winners and losers. Do not make it personal.

If you struggle to do yourself justice in these situations, invest in a course that teaches interview skills. It is likely to cost you a couple of hundred pounds and will give you a foundation on which you can build. You will face interviews in a variety of forms along the way. If you can overcome some of your fears at this stage, it will be money well spent. If you feel that you generally cope well with an interview situation, you may not need to go on a formal course, but you should still get someone, ideally a consultant (or two if possible, as this will make it more realistic), to give you some mock interviews. This is a good rehearsal to assess the impact of the answers you have prepared. Are you pitching them at the right level or do you become tongue-tied when you try? Do they sound too rehearsed? This works well as a means of getting some constructive criticism and gives you an idea of what the real thing will be like.

Interview panels are generally amenable and genuinely trying to find out if you are what they are looking for rather than trying to intimidate you. They aim to relax candidates as much as possible so that each can show themselves in the best light. However, you are bound to find it stressful (as will all the other candidates), but since you will be working in conditions that will bring on stress at times, it is not inappropriate that your panel get a chance to see how you respond. This is very different from trying to bully or intimidate information from you. The usual mantras ring true – dress appropriately, adopt an air of cheerful optimism and quiet confidence, and try to make your body language as well as your verbal statements positive. Perhaps hardest of all – if you feel you have made a mistake or could have done better – do not give up. Put it behind you and answer the next question as best you can. Very few people have a perfect interview – keep going and you may salvage it.

Once it is over, listen to the instructions. If you are going to be informed of the outcome that day, do not go and get drunk before the announcement – the difficult bit may be over but you may be called upon to make an important decision in choosing a rotation. There was one famous set of interviews where a series of candidates turned down precious National Training Numbers because of the restrictions attached – such as having to leave research posts early and therefore sacrifice the prospect of finishing their thesis. Declining a job under these circumstances takes some nerve and is not an easy decision and would be impossible to judge adequately after a few pints. Wait until the very end before you celebrate.

You Got the Job!

You should, quite rightly, be thrilled – congratulations! It is important that you check what you are lined up for. Try to find out where you are starting and contact the department there. Go and see the consultants, armed with a CV – this makes contact with them so they know whom they are getting and your baseline experience and sets you on the right road. Speak to human resources early – get your health checks done and make sure all your registration details are in order (this is your responsibility and it is no good trying to blame occupational health on the day you start – you should know what is expected of you). If you are unsure about your salary scale, take advice – if you are a member of the BMA, they can be very helpful. Despite this being common sense, it is not commonly sorted out – people somehow expect this all to be done for them – it will not!

While You Are Waiting

It is natural that you will feel out of phase with clinical work – especially if you have been primarily working in a lab for 2 or 3 years. It may be that your own specialty organization runs a clinical skills course that you could attend to re-familiarize yourself. Go and shadow a colleague – see what they do. Sit in a few clinics with one of the consultants in your current department and refresh your memory. This will make you look and feel less like a complete novice in your first clinic with your new consultant. If you are likely to use complex equipment go and spend sometime with the nurses or other staff who will be using it with you. Get them to go through how you take it apart and put it back together – this will earn the respect of the theater staff before you have even set foot in the door. Both you and they will have some confidence that you will not to look a complete fool the first time you come to pick up an instrument and use it.

Table 10.1 Getting back

Keep a plan for your future career in mind
Obtain an application form for your next post early in research
Confirm that you have all essential criteria
Achieve as many desirable criteria as possible
Prepare thoroughly for interview, and consider an interview skills course to get back up to date quickly
Reintroduce yourself to more clinical work toward the end of the project but do not let this detract from finishing off your thesis!

In your excitement of preparing to reenter clinical practice, do not forget that it is vital that you get your research finished and as close to written up as possible.

In summary, you will have to grin and bear any application process that exists when you come to apply. The key is preparation, both in terms of short-listing and interview. While you wait to start your job – WRITE UP YOUR THESIS. It is useful to go to some clinics and operating lists before you start to try and refresh your clinical memory. Do not get too carried away – all this will follow when you are back in the clinical setting – your priority remains to *WRITE UP YOUR THESIS*! (Table 10.1).

Chapter 11
Life After…

For a chapter summary, see Table 11.1.

Your approach to this period in your life will depend entirely on how successful your time in research has been and therefore how you feel about it. If you have not got any results, had no money, or suffered through either a lack of supervision or conflict with your supervisor, it would require the rosiest of rose tinted spectacles to believe that you have had a positive research experience. If things have been better than this, then you may well be considering your options. You may well feel that you have done your time, gained as much as you can from research, and be preparing to move on to develop other areas – this is the case for the vast majority of people. Alternatively, you may wish to try to continue with research. There is now a more formalized career structure for achieving this – there are the academic training numbers and it is envisioned that this will offer a dedicated career path for those wishing to pursue an academic career. At the time of writing, relatively few have been appointed and it remains to be seen how this process will work in the long term. If you are only able to use your (nominal) academic half day to do research, you are likely to find that this is insufficient to do any hands on work and therefore to sustain your previous

D. Smith, D. Wood, *Research in Clinical Practice,*
DOI 10.1007/978-1-4471-2873-1_11,
© Springer-Verlag London 2013

progress. Even if you discuss this with your training committee, they may feel that you have been appointed first and foremost as a specialist registrar and that this should be your primary commitment. In addition, funding opportunities to maintain your research interest may also be few and far between, particularly if your subject area is not currently "in vogue," such as molecular biology or oncological heroism, and hence does not easily attract funding.

If you aim to pursue a career in academic medicine or you discover that continuing research would be something you have unexpectedly decided to pursue, then discuss these ideas early and try to obtain an academic training number – this will fast become the established route for your new-found career path.

What to Do If You Have Not Written Up...

You may have already gathered that this is an appalling situation to be in. Many friends and colleagues have been in this position – for a variety of reasons ranging from having been unable to get data early on to having to change direction and therefore running out of time, weak supervision, poor turn around (by supervisors) of thesis drafts (6–8 months was the case for some), or simply through a lack of personal application and self-direction. Without doubt, this is your project and it is you that will be judged on the completion of your thesis or not – it is unlikely to reflect too much on anybody else. Even though there may be elements that are out of your control, you need to try to avoid the scenario of writing up after your research period is over as this is, quite simply, a nightmare. From the time you rejoin a clinical job until the time you finally hand in a thesis, it will hang over you, depress you and your trainers, and not only your supervisor but also your family will nag you about it.

The best solution is to realize early on that the above situation is one to be avoided and therefore to work hard to get your thesis written up while you are still in whole-time research. Those who do end up in this position are constantly frustrated by evenings spent reading, editing, and reediting half written chapters; falling asleep before making any progress; and weekends divided between a young family and data analysis. In fact, you will likely have to use some of your annual leave as it is impossible to remember your thought process and pick these up again in a meaningful way on the odd evening or weekend. You need to take a week or two in order to make any significant headway. In these circumstances, it requires an enormous amount of personal resolve and drive to complete a thesis – it takes about 3 years after finishing research for most, compared with 3–6 months while you are still in the protected environment of research. If this is the timescale, once the thesis is finished, many will have to launch straight into work for their specialty exit exam – misery. Although training committees may allow you to take a couple of months sabbatical in order to complete, not only is this financially an expensive option but it may also delay your CCT (Certificate of Completion of Training) date. However, as the requirements for appointments tighten, it may well be that if you were appointed on the basis of working towards a thesis that you will not be granted your CCT without successfully completing your thesis – so beware!

The bottom line, therefore, is do not end up here. Complete writing up *before* your research time is up, so you can then enjoy your clinical work, write a few clinical papers, and get the most out of your training. You also avoid impinging on your family life with your thesis forevermore.

If you have not done the work by this stage, then you have only yourself to blame and it is only you that can sort it out. If you are having other problems, you must discuss them. If your supervisor is taking an excessive time to get your draft sections back to you, start by talking to them. As we have said before, it is often better to manage this by giving in sections rather than the whole book at once. This means that you can be working away at other sections while he or she looks at what you have given in – this minimizes delay. It is good to be around while you are writing up so that you can check in and ask how they are getting on with what you have given them – just a gentle shove in the right direction. If you are not in the lab anymore, then you can always send polite reminders by e-mail.

Ultimately, if your supervisor is not moving at the pace you were hoping for, you must address it with them. Remember there are two sides to every story so just ensure that you are not being impractical with your expectations and consider that your supervisor may be very busy. See if there are ways that you can make their life easier. If it is a persistent problem, then you need to try to say something about how it is worrying you and why you feel there is a pressure to move on (training committee, etc.). After all, your failure to complete looks bad for them too, not least as anyone who has read this book will now seek out your supervisor to ask how many theses get written up and what level of support research fellows get in the lab. It may even mean that they struggle to recruit in future and worse that they struggle to get grants if their fellows do not complete their projects.

If the problem is not resolved by a direct discussion, you should involve an alternative supervisor (e.g., a clinical supervisor): even if they have not been particularly involved up to this point, they can now be your savior. It is not ideal to alienate people, so a constructive approach involving an explanation of the difficulties to both supervisors and trying to find the best solution between you is likely to be the best for you. There may be occasions when a supervisor is inadvertently more obstructive than helpful or creates confusion by offering very different opinions or lacking consistency. In these situations, you may have to find someone else to help you submit your thesis. If so, you must be certain that they have the necessary standing within the university to allow them to sign your submission papers, etc., before you terminate the relationship with your main supervisor.

Looking from the other perspective, if your supervisor objects strongly to your data or conclusions, they can seek to distance themselves from your work (via an established university mechanism) and in this situation that may actually be to your benefit – providing you have alternative support.

In any event, you should keep your clinical supervisors appraised of the situation. They may be able to help and will be more able to accommodate your dilemmas if you are honest and open. People do not generally appreciate surprises in these situations – avoid them if possible.

Papers, Presentations, etc.

Towards the end of your research, you will (hopefully) have a few presentations to make and one or two papers to publish. This is very exciting but requires a degree of balance to ensure you do not spend your whole time going to meetings and never doing any real work.

Posters

Many people see posters as something of a lesser option as far as meetings are concerned. It is unlikely that you will have your name in lights for a plenary session at your first international conference. You are most likely to present at a poster session. These can be great sessions and, depending on the meeting, may be attended by significant figures within your field.

Contact your medical illustration department early – there are often instructions about what they need from you on the web. Agree your format with supervisors and coauthors and allow yourself time to put things together and revise them. This may take several weeks, and bearing in mind that your poster is likely to have been accepted months beforehand, this should not be too much of a pressure.

Ideally, when you collect your poster do so a week or so before you travel, which gives you time to correct mistakes (if necessary). All of the above is the counsel of perfection and although it sounds simple, it can be remarkably difficult to achieve.

It is worth attending a similar session to your own in advance, so that you can familiarize yourself with the format of the room and of the likely dynamics of the session. When it comes to your turn, follow the instructions and remember the chairman is your friend. If they ask you to summarize your main conclusions in 2 min, then do exactly this. A surprising number of people feel that this is an invitation to share the details of their life's work to this point. A good chairman will aim to keep a session moving, stimulate questions of interest, and protect the presenter from unreasonable questioning. In the interests of other presenters and the session overall, if you do not comply with the requests of your chairman, it is likely that you will be sped along or even asked to stop. If this happens, not only will you feel daft, you may lose your nerve or concentration for questions. In this regard, if you do not know the answer to a question – say so as there may be people in the audience who do know and who will not be impressed by your obvious attempts to disguise your missing knowledge and you will end up doing yourself a disservice.

Be prepared for people to stop at your poster and want to ask you questions – these conversations can be extremely interesting and productive. In general, those people doing this will have a genuine interest and may also have helpful suggestions as to how you might continue with your work. Your chairmen will also attempt to meet you and ask you about your work – this is a good chance to try to assess their views and perhaps gauge any likely questions for the main session.

At the end of the session, write down all of the questions that were raised about your work, both at the poster and in the presentation of it, especially any suggestions for future research that were made. You can use these to guide further experiments or as ideas to explore in your discussion.

Papers

However long you think this will take, treble it and then treble it again. We all have aspirations to see our names in *Nature* and anticipate that we will write that paper over the course of the next week. This never happens. Collecting data, even at the height of productivity, takes weeks or months, and analyzing it takes several weeks more. Writing your first draft will also take weeks, at which point your senior authors will pull it to pieces and you will begin again. Hopefully over a reasonably short time, you will be close to a final version that you then submit. Review processes vary enormously between journals but when you get comments back, try to turn them around as soon as possible. It would be totally inappropriate for this book to attempt to give you a comprehensive guide to writing your paper – there are many books and courses on the subject and it is worth taking in one or more of these, but practice is the key and the more you publish, the more you will get published.

Many people have published enthusiastically and relent-lessly. The most credible authors are those that make good use of data in focused publications. From your own perspective, this offers the best chance of achieving publication in a journal of note rather than one that could be considered a less significant publication. There are different ways of judging the importance of a journal. The most established and accepted form is the impact factor or citation index. This is a measure of how often work from a journal is cited in subsequent litera-ture – the principle being that the more your work is cited the better it is. Hence, the higher the impact factor for a journal, the more highly it is regarded academically, and in measuring the success of institutions and departments, this is very impor-tant. Clearly, this is important at an individual level too but there is room for discretion. There is little point in publishing your latest surgical technique in a journal that will not be read by a relevant audience, so it also important to consider this in deciding where you will submit. Reformatting can be time consuming so discuss your target journal early, with other authors, and make a realistic plan your publication.

Maintaining Links

You have to hope that when you finally lay down your last test tube and leave the lab that you will have enjoyed your time and gained something worthwhile from the whole exercise.

There may well be things that you still need to complete with the lab – namely, papers and your thesis! You may decide that you wish to continue your interest further. As noted previously, this is probably best achieved through an academic training number unless you only want to pursue it on an informal basis. Either way, you should express your interest and try to establish a way of achieving your goals. You will have to be realistic about how much you can achieve and contribute but you may well have useful additions to make, and in the long term, you may continue to gain from the relationship. You may also have a useful role in other aspects for the lab such as getting tissue specimens or encouraging new researchers to enter the lab – this makes your continued relationship with the lab mutually important.

Closing Remarks

One of the most astute remarks about research is that it teaches you to deal with disappointment. You will regularly encounter difficulties and frustrations; there will be days when you want to give it all up and leave – there will be days when you feel that is only a matter of time before the Nobel Academy come knocking at your door (though these are far less common!). Part of undertaking research is to be able to deal with both aspects of your work – as in Rudyard Kipling's great poem:

> If you can meet with triumph and disaster
> And treat those two imposters just the same

Moving up in clinical medicine offers similar highs and lows in your day to day practice – in this environment, you have to learn how to deal with these difficulties and cope with success all in a professional way. Some of the skills you acquire in research will undoubtedly stand you in good stead for these situations.

All doctors have a responsibility to maintain their own standards both in clinical practice and education – there is no doubt that time in research helps with this enormously as you

Table 11.1 Life after

Make sure your thesis is completed as soon as possible
Give a section to your supervisor to approve while you work on the next
Go to meetings and raise your profile
Write a paper (or two)
Keep in touch with your research colleagues, especially your supervisor – even if you are not planning more research, you may change your mind or want your own research fellow one day

will not achieve anything significant without an approach that requires attention to detail. While we do not believe that all doctors should have to undertake research, we do believe that a period of insight into research and its importance for the development of medicine as a whole should be incorporated into every training program. For those of you who are pursuing a full-time research commitment (and that may be all of you who have reached this far), we close by wishing you a fruitful and fulfilling time in your endeavors (Table 11.1).

Good Luck!

Index

D. Smith, D. Wood, *Research in Clinical Practice,*
DOI 10.1007/978-1-4471-2873-1,
© Springer-Verlag London 2013